I0073843

Carpal Tunnel Syndrome, CTS explained.

Carpal Tunnel Syndrome causes, symptoms, treatment, exercises, management, therapies and prevention.

by

Lucy Rudford

ALL RIGHTS RESERVED. This book contains material protected under International and Federal Copyright Laws and Treaties.

Any unauthorized reprint or use of this material is strictly prohibited.

No part of this book may be reproduced or transmitted in any form or by any means, electronic, mechanical or otherwise, including photocopying or recording, or by any information storage and retrieval system without express written permission from the author.

Copyrighted © 2014

Published by: IMB Publishing

Table of Contents

Table of Contents

Table of Contents

Table of Contents

Table of Contents

Foreword

As many as one in fifty patients are believed to suffer from Carpal Tunnel Syndrome, with a significant percentage of those patients suffering a worsening of their symptoms over time.

Many patients with this nerve entrapment will suffer from bilateral Carpal Tunnel Syndrome, meaning that the condition will affect both hands.

While there are many treatment options available, there are some arguments over the most effective course of treatment, so this book clearly lays out all of the options that are available to patients from diagnosis to conventional treatments and natural alternatives and exercises. The book also provides many helpful, practical tips aimed at preventing the onset of Carpal Tunnel Syndrome.

Throughout this book, the patient will be encouraged to look at the various treatments available and find an effective programme of therapy or therapies to help themselves.

This book explains to the patient how to treat Carpal Tunnel Syndrome and puts the power in the patient's hands as well as helping them to discover the measures they can take to help themselves, while gaining a greater understanding of the condition.

As Carpal Tunnel Syndrome (CTS) is very often caused by Repetitive Strain Injury (RSI) by overuse of computers, I will also talk about RSI injuries in this book and about the importance of working correctly on a computer. The majority of Carpal Tunnel Sufferers work in an office environment.

I am going to tell you the most important things you need to know to prevent Carpal Tunnel Syndrome all together or to prevent it from coming back if you have already suffered from it.

There are three things that I encourage absolutely everybody to do whilst texting, working on a pc a laptop/tablet or playing on a game console:

* **TAKE REGULAR BREAKS**

* **DO REGULAR EXERCISES** e.g. stretch your neck, arms and back

* **MAKE SURE YOU ARE SITTING IN THE CORRECT POSITION** whilst on your PC or laptop (not on your bed with your laptop on your lap) and if you can afford it, buy an ergonomic chair.

I hope that my book not only helps you to prevent CTS but also helps you to deal with it.

It is no joke, really, please take this seriously and look after your future health. You will read sufferer's stories throughout this book.

Make sure not to become a sufferer with a story yourself, if it is not already too late.

Don't ignore your symptoms as it really comes down to this one simple message:

ACT NOW

OR

SUFFER FOREVER!

You will find sufferer's stories in Italics in this book. These are REAL stories from REAL sufferers. The aim of these is clear: to make you, the reader, understand how badly Carpal Tunnel Syndrome can influence every day life.

Introduction

Carpal Tunnel Syndrome is a relatively common condition that causes pain and, in some advanced cases, disability. In this book, the reader will learn exactly what Carpal Tunnel Syndrome is and what can be done about it.

The reader will discover the different treatment options such as physiotherapy, the use of carpal tunnel splints, and the types of medication that are available to patients. The different kinds of surgery will also be explained.

This book aims to explain all of the different treatments available to patients. This includes exercises and tools to maintain dexterity and to prevent muscle loss, the different types of natural therapies that are available to try, and natural remedies that have been shown to be helpful for some patients.

This book also explores the wider picture and encourages the patient to not just concentrate on the Carpal Tunnel Syndrome itself, but all of the factors that contribute to it such as poor posture, overuse, hand position etc. The book will also detail the many other conditions that can affect the upper body, helping the reader to come up with an effective plan to manage those symptoms too.

For those with advanced symptoms, there is practical advice that explains the kinds of tools that are available to help patients with Carpal Tunnel Syndrome maintain their dexterity and independence, and there is also advice on how patients can access the help that they need.

This book also explains the importance of ensuring that people have a healthy workspace in order to help prevent or reduce the symptoms of this painful condition.

Most importantly, this book is full of hints and tips to help patients realise that there is plenty they can do to help themselves.

Patients will also learn the importance of the role occupational therapists can play in helping patients recover from surgery, how they can design their workspace so as to lessen their chances of developing Carpal Tunnel Syndrome, and a qualified occupational therapist will explain the kind of help that is available to help people return to work if they have a history of Carpal Tunnel Syndrome.

Throughout the book, the importance of keeping the patient's medical team informed of what they are doing – or what they plan to do – is stressed so that their medical team can discuss the advantages and possible disadvantages of taking a particular course of action. Severe Carpal Tunnel Syndrome will often require surgery, so the various surgical techniques are also explained.

Above all, this book sets out to empower the reader so that they know that there is plenty that they can do to help themselves by addressing their symptoms one by one and learning to manage them more effectively.

Sufferer's Story: *Four years ago I developed a repetitive strain injury in both hands, wrists, arms, shoulders and neck. The vagus nerve was affected and after 15 minutes of doing any kind of work with my arms - washing up, driving, writing, working on the computer - I was in tears from the sickening, aching pain. The hospital physiotherapist told me I presented the most severe and extensive case she had ever seen and warned me I was unlikely to recover fully. I spent hundreds of pounds each month visiting chiropractors, osteopaths and massage therapists, and although they all provided some relief, nothing lasted. I began to wonder if I could ever work again.* Source: www.stat.org.uk

Statistics and facts:

As Carpal Tunnel Syndrome (CTS) is very often caused by Repetitive Strain Injury (RSI), I will also incluse RSI statistics and facts.

- Six people in the UK leave their jobs every day due to RSI.

- Over half of adults in the U.S. reported a musculoskeletal condition in 2009. Source: Centres for Disease Control and Prevention.

- Ten percent of the sick notes written in London are for RSIs. Source: -London Evening Standard

- From 2004 to 2012, managing musculoskeletal diseases, including lost wages, cost an average $850 billion each year. Source: U.S. Department of Health.

- Office ergonomics training can reduce the average cost per workers' compensation claims by 90 percent, according to at least one study. Source: International Journal of Industrial Ergonomics Claims Management Company www.antriumlegal.com

- 30 percent of frequent computer users complain of tingling, burning or numbness of limbs. Source: American Family Physician

- 10 percent of frequent computer users have carpal tunnel syndrome, which is just one of many different types of RSIs. Source: American Family Physician

- In 2006, 450,000 workers in the UK (that's nearly one out of every 50 workers) reported RSIs. Source: Chartered Society of Physiotherapy

- British workers lost 3.5 million working days from RSIs in 2006-07 alone, at a cost of between £300 million. Source: Chartered Society of Physiotherapy

- Musculoskeletal disorders and diseases are the leading cause of disability in the United States and account for more than 50 percent of all chronic conditions in people over 50 years of age in developed countries. Source: American Academy of Orthopaedic Surgeons

- One out of every 50 workers in the UK have reported symptoms of RSIs. Source: Repetitive Strain Injury Association.

- 5.4 million working days are lost due to RSIs every year in the UK. Source: Repetitive Strain Injury Association.

- 45 percent of Irish workers have experienced RSI. Source: Siliconrepublic.com

www.repetitivestraininjuryhelp.com says:

- Globally, the most conventional approximation of related cost of repetitive strain injury disorders run into thousands of millions of dollars.

- Approximately, 63% of all office employees spend their most of time in holding mouse than any other device.

- More than 100 million individuals worldwide are predicted to suffer from some type of RSI or other computer associated health problems.

- According to recent surveys, insufficient breaks while working on system are the key factors responsible for encouraging the development of repetitive strain injury.

- RSI is unlikely to develop in single form, in several reports it has been established that the combination of lots of factors contribute to the repetitive strain injury risks.

- Taking regular breaks from working and releasing pressure on forearms, wrists and hands has seemed beneficial.

- The efficacy of most of preventative measures and ergonomics are disputed. No researches have presented these measures to be effectual in avoiding repetitive strain injury so far.

Cost involved in preventing RSI - according to www.repetitivestraininjuryhelp.com:

Now-a-days, a huge amount of money is being invested in avoiding the risk of RSI as governments and employees have been becoming aware of the widespread effects of this problem. Several RSI research studies suggest that ergonomic is one of the helpful ways to prevent RSI. They have also established that for every one dollar spent in RSI prevention, there is a return of approximately 17 dollars. A wide variety of ergonomics has been introduced ranging from armrests to keyboards costing about 100 dollars to other complete ergonomics desktops costing thousands of dollars.

It is really very difficult to figure out the exact amount that the government of a nation spends on preventing RSI. In the UK, almost 8 to 30 million USD have invested in treatment or preventing RSI while in the USA, this amount goes to 40 million USD. In the European Union, about 40 to 60 millions USD are spent on RSI.

Chapter 1) Carpal Tunnel Syndrome

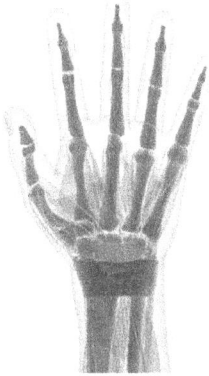

1) What is the Carpal Tunnel?

The carpal tunnel is found on the palm side of the wrist. The carpal tunnel is effectively a passageway where several nerves and tendons pass through. There are several flexor tendons in the carpal (wrist) tunnel and the tunnel is made up of bones from the wrist. When one or more of these tendons gets swollen through injury, overuse or disease it can cause the tunnel to narrow.

The Carpal Tunnel

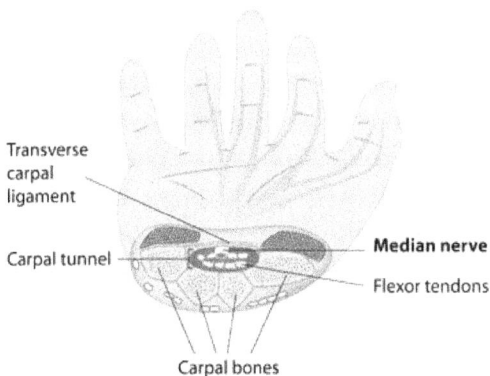

Transverse carpal ligament

Carpal tunnel

Median nerve

Flexor tendons

Carpal bones

2) What is Carpal Tunnel Syndrome?

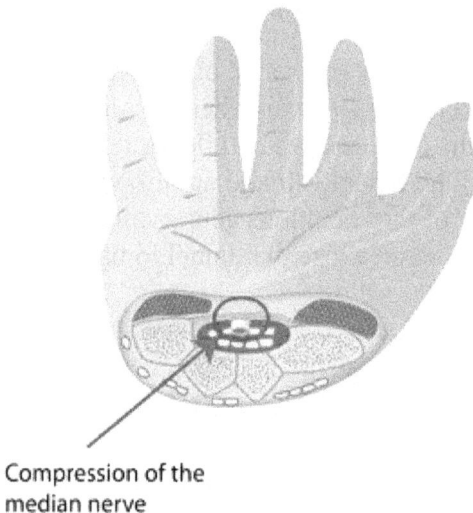

In addition to the tendons, there are several nerves that run into the carpal tunnel. When the tendons are swollen or injured, they can then entrap the median nerve, which is located in the wrist. It is when this nerve becomes entrapped or compressed that the symptoms of Carpal Tunnel Syndrome begin.

Carpal Tunnel Syndrome can often be the result of a repetitive action such as typing or using tools or it can be caused by sudden trauma to the wrist such as a sprain or a fracture. Patients with an underlying medical condition can also be vulnerable to Carpal Tunnel Syndrome; patients with arthritis, diabetes and low thyroid all have a greater prevalence of CTS.

Carpal Tunnel Syndrome

Compression of the
median nerve

3) Carpal Tunnel Syndrome - symptoms

When the median nerve becomes entrapped, patients can begin to experience motor and sensory symptoms. The signs of Carpal Tunnel Syndrome might not be noticeable at first. Sensory symptoms include pain, tingling in the fingers, with the exception of the little finger, numbness, pain and feelings of the hand going to sleep; some people also wake up with a numb feeling in their arm. An early sign of Carpal Tunnel Syndrome might be tingling in the arm after a long time spent typing. Symptoms of Carpal Tunnel Syndrome might also occur after an accident or injury.

Signs of Carpal Tunnel Syndrome might go un-noticed at first as they are often minor. This can sometimes mean that the patient will have had Carpal Tunnel Syndrome for a long time before being diagnosed, which can make treatment more complex as the symptoms will have been allowed to worsen.

As the symptoms can also come on slowly, the patient is likely to continue with the same actions that have caused their condition without realising that anything is wrong.

The pain is most often felt in the wrist area and in the fingers, however, some patients might also experience discomfort in their lower arm, shoulder and neck.

In addition, some patients with Carpal Tunnel Syndrome can go on to develop motor symptoms. This can mean a loss of strength, problems gripping and clumsiness due to the inability to grasp hold of objects properly.

Sufferer's story: *"... my partner is desperately bored of my symptoms and finds me exceptionally annoying - and useless! He tells me to shut up 'cos he knows what I'm about to say - I'm a broken record. If he catches me having a whimper upstairs he rants and raves at me to grow up, change my job, get an operation. Although I would appreciate his sympathy occasionally I sort of understand where he's coming from - it must be tedious to have someone whining [sic]away doing the most mundane of chores!"* Source: Watson, M. 2009. Investigating the experiences of people with RSI. http://etheses.qmu.ac.uk/133/

RSIs are more common than most people think.

RSIs are progressive: they get worse over time and they rarely get better on their own. They can, however, be treated. If you recognise the symptoms early, you can get treatment before you become disabled. The sooner you start treatment, the more successful the treatment is likely to be.

When you first notice symptoms, unfortunately you have already done substantial damage to your body.

Symptoms of the different types of RSIs differ, but there are a number of typical early RSI indicators. Many RSI suffers find that symptoms come and go seemingly without explanation because they develop gradually, often over a long period of time, so the early symptoms are often overlooked.

a) Early signs
- Aches, pains, cramps, swelling or tenderness in muscles or joints. Pain may be mild or severe; it may be burning or shooting. You may feel pain in specific locations like your fingers or you may feel it along your entire arm and hand. Pain may move and be hard to pinpoint. You may have pain in areas of the body distant from the site of the injury e.g. you may get a pain in your upper neck but the real problem is in the muscle of your lower neck.

- Fatigue. Sufferers may get tired from activities they could previously do for long periods of time without difficulty.

- Headaches. If you get the headaches only when you are doing your repetitive movements, it could be a sign that some muscles in your neck are not working properly. Headaches on top of your head or on one side of your head (left or right forehead) are often a sign of damage to certain muscles. Trigger point massage or deep tissue can be very helpful for this.

- Weakness of the arms. Weakness can make it hard to do simple tasks. When weakness affects grip strength, sufferers may need two hands to hold onto objects.

- Restricted movement of limbs. Difficulty opening and closing your hands or using your hands for normal activities.

- **Cold hands.** Cold hands can indicate nerve damage.

- **Hypersensitivity.** A light touch over a strained muscle or tendon may feel painful.

- **Reduced sensation**. On the other end of the spectrum from hypersensitivity is diminished feeling in the fingers.

b) Later symptoms
- **Numbness and/or tingling**. When hands often feel like they have fallen asleep it may be a sign of nerve damage.

- **Spasms, tremors, and/or twitching in the forearms**.

- **Continuous pain in the affected area, even without movement**. The pain may be severe enough to wake the RSI sufferer up during the night.

- **Difficulty holding onto objects.** When the arms and hands become weaker, sufferers may find themselves dropping simple objects like coffee cups or pens. They may not have the strength to pick up a sack of groceries or even hold onto a child.

c) Continuum of Symptoms
In their book Repetitive Strain Injury: A Computer User's Guide, Dr. Emil Pascarelli and Deborah Quilter outline a continuum of RSI that describes the symptoms and the typical course of untreated RSIs:

- **Pre-RSI:** "Funny" feeling in arms or hands, relieved by rest.

- **Early RSI**: Intermittent pain or tingling while typing, relieved by rest and rehabilitation.

- **Danger Zone**: Weakness, clumsiness, intermittent pain not necessarily relieved by rest; daily activities impaired; depression. Moderate risk of permanent impairment.

- **Chronic Pain:** Weakness, constant pain, not relieved by rest and made worse by any activity. High risk of permanent impairment and disability.

- **Chronic Pain and Dysfunction:** Chronic pain; depression, dystonia (painful involuntary contractions of the muscles); severe chronic pain with weakness, tremors, and spasms. Permanent disability.

d) Changes in Habits

RSI sufferers may change their habits or make excuses for their symptoms without even knowing it. They may start using paper plates so they don't risk dropping dishes. Or, they may change sports, like taking up jogging instead of playing tennis as they used to. They may say they can't pick up the baby because their back hurts. They may stop wearing neckties, saying they prefer the casual look when in reality it's because they can no longer knot their ties. People who suffer from RSI may not realize that they are changing their lives to accommodate their injuries but they should be changing their lives to prevent them.

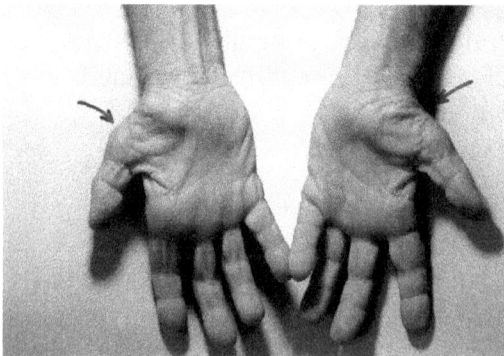

Untreated Carpal Tunnel Syndrome Source :
http://upload.wikimedia.org/wikipedia/commons/thumb/6/68/Untr
eated_Carpal_Tunnel_Syndrome.JPG/1024px-
Untreated_Carpal_Tunnel_Syndrome.JPG

4) Bi-Lateral Carpal Tunnel Syndrome

Bi-Lateral Carpal Tunnel Syndrome simply means that the condition affects both wrists. While some experts argue that this form of entrapment neuropathy most often affects just one side, one study has shown that it is likely that many patients do in fact have CTS in both hands; it is just that the symptoms are more noticeable on one side.

However, the study also states that the symptoms of CTS can worsen over time, thus causing the common signs of CTS to become more noticeable.

5) Carpal Tunnel Syndrome – Diagnosis

Sometimes a doctor won't deem it necessary to send a patient for further tests to determine whether or not they have a nerve entrapment.

A family doctor can often make a diagnosis just by listening to the symptoms the patient describes. If a GP suspects that the patient does have CTS then the first step will be to prescribe anti-inflammatory medication.

There is a Carpal Tunnel Syndrome test that might be used to diagnose CTS; it's called the Tinel test. During the Tinel test, the doctor will press on the median nerve. If this causes discomfort such as pain or tingling in the fingers, then it will be considered a sign that the patient does indeed have Carpal Tunnel Syndrome.

Another test, the Phalen Test, where the wrist is held in a flexed position, might also be applied.

If further diagnosis is required, the patients will be referred to a consultant neurologist at the nearest hospital. There are two tests that can be carried out to further assess the condition. The first is a nerve conduction test. This will measure how well the nerve impulses are working. The test will tell the neurologist whether there is nerve damage or nerve injury.

The second is called an electromyography or an EMG. This will show how well the muscles are working by recording the electrical activity in the muscles. EMGs are commonly used to diagnose conditions such as neuropathy, nerve damage and Carpal Tunnel Syndrome.

Another way of diagnosing CTS is by the use of ultrasonography. Ultrasonography uses ultrasound technology to determine what is going on inside the body's structure. Although this isn't one of the most commonly used methods of testing for the presence of CTS, studies have shown that it an effective means of diagnosing the condition.

6) What Causes Carpal Tunnel Syndrome?

There is no single cause for CTS, but there are factors that increase the risk for injury. Risk factors are events or conditions that increase the likelihood of a disorder occurring, but are not necessarily the cause. **Basically anybody who carries out the same movement over and over for years and years is at risk.**

The risk factors for CTS/RSI include:

a) Poorly designed workstations or tools.

b) Working for long periods of time without enough breaks.

c) Repetitive movements

- holding one's phone between neck and shoulder all day

- carrying heavy items

- texting all day long

- sitting in the same position for too long

- using a laptop for hours without breaks

- working on a PC for hours without a break

RSI-sufferers story: "*Doctors have disagreed with each other, and blamed each other for not doing the right thing. My employers don't know what to believe. I feel like my employers have written me off. My doctor told me to hang my job up. That's a huge decision.*" Source: Repetitive Strain Injury: A Computer User's Guide by Emil Pascarelli, MD and Deborah Quilter.

There are a number of causes of Carpal Tunnel Syndrome. Listed below are some of the common causes:

- Diabetes

- Arthritis

- Hypothyroid

- Pregnancy

- Injury

- Trauma

- Repetitive Stress

a) Diabetes
Patients with type one or type two diabetes are more susceptible to Carpal Tunnel Syndrome and other forms of nerve damage such as neuropathy.

Patients with diabetes experiencing symptoms of numbness or tingling in their fingers or pain in the wrist area should visit their doctor or raise their concerns with their diabetes consultant who can refer them for further tests if required.

b) Arthritis
Arthritis is another common cause of CTS. The syndrome is often associated with bone and joint diseases and swelling in the wrist

area could contribute to the development of Carpal Tunnel Syndrome.

c) Hypothyroidism

Hypothyroidism is common in patients with diabetes and this can mean that people being treated for diabetes have an increased chance of developing Carpal Tunnel Syndrome.

Having low thyroid function can leave patients more likely to develop tendon problems, which could play a role in the development of Carpal Tunnel Syndrome, however, many studies have been carried out and there has been no clear causative link found.

d) Carpal Tunnel Syndrome -Pregnancy

Some women develop Carpal Tunnel Syndrome in pregnancy. The reasons for this are not completely clear, however, it is believed that the disruption in the hormone balance can contribute to this by causing swelling and fluid retention. Any woman experiencing the symptoms of Carpal Tunnel Syndrome during pregnancy should talk to their doctor rather than trying to manage the symptoms themselves.

The hormonal link might also explain why some women are more prone to developing CTS.

e) Injury and Trauma

Any injury or trauma to the wrist area that causes swelling or tendon damage can cause a compression on the median nerve, which can go on to develop into Carpal Tunnel Syndrome.

f) Repetitive Stress

Repetitive Stress is perhaps the most common cause of Carpal Tunnel Syndrome. Repetitive Stress Injury or Work Related Upper Body Disorder, as it is now more commonly known, does not just occur in people who do a lot of typing work.

RSI is also common in dentists, musicians, builders and bakers. Paul Hollywood, the baker now best known for his role in *The Great British Bake Off* announced last year that his years of rolling dough had led to him developing numbness in his hands as a result of his profession.

Another common cause of repetitive stress injury is the high prevalence of hand held gadgets and mobile phones. People who spend a lot of time texting, playing games on hand held devices or repeatedly pressing keys can go on to develop Carpal Tunnel Syndrome due to the repetitive nature of these actions.

People who like to spend a lot of time playing computer games are also more likely to go on to develop Carpal Tunnel Syndrome as a result of the overuse of the tendons, which will ultimately lead to swelling and inflammation.

"The Blackberry Thumb", as a result of too much typing on mobile devices, is a frequently talked about topic amongst doctors and chiropractors. Now "text neck" is added to their vocabulary and is causing symptoms like neck strain, shoulder pain, headaches, and pain the arms and hands.

RSIs can develop gradually over weeks, months, even years. Symptoms may come and go, making them difficult to pinpoint and even harder to diagnose. By the time they get to the doctor, people may be suffering from shooting pains, numb fingers, and muscle spasms. Due to the fact that their pain and limitations are invisible, people who suffer from RSIs may be seen as lazy and unwilling to do their share of the work.

For a long time, RSIs were found almost exclusively amongst workers who did physical work, especially cleaners, cooks, meatpackers, machine operators, and construction workers. When personal computers appeared on the desks of office workers in the 1980s, RSIs expanded into the office workforce. With the explosive popularity of computers for personal use, such as cell phones, PDAs, game consoles, and other electronic devices, RSIs have spread into the general population. Research in Sweden found that one-half of the people who work with computers have pains in their necks, shoulders, arms, or hands.

There's another change in the population at risk: RSIs are no longer found only amongst adults. As young people participate more and more in the new technologies, growing numbers of children and teenagers are reporting aches, pains, and discomfort when using their computers, mobile phones, and video game consoles.

Attracted by the colours and images, even toddlers are drawn to computers. The long-term consequences for early computer users are not yet known, but medical experts fear that we may be raising generations of young adults who start their work lives already injured. What will happen as they age is the great unknown. Will they be able to work? Enjoy hobbies? Hold their children?

This is a BIG problem in this modern electronic society.

RSIs and the subsequent Carpal Tunnel Sydrome take a huge toll on individuals, affecting their jobs, financial stability, enjoyment of life, and personal relationships. The impaired functioning that can result in job loss also affects activities of daily living, such as carrying groceries, lifting a child, or dressing one's self. It is not uncommon for RSI sufferers to be unable to button their shirts or to tie their own shoes. Their social lives diminish as they become less and less able to participate in pleasurable activities. Depression, anger, frustration and low self-esteem may accompany the pain and disability of RSIs. As one 35-year-old woman lamented: *"...RSI has destroyed my carefully built up confidence. I used to be a pretty happy person most of the time. I feel that I've permanently lost that person."*

g) Obesity

Studies have indicated that being obese can leave a patient more vulnerable to Carpal Tunnel Syndrome. Although further research is needed, it has been shown that patients who lose weight experience a lessening of their symptoms; however the research indicated that there could also be other factors that will be contributing to the CTS, rather than just the excess weight.

Chapter 2) Is This Your Future?

The truth hurts! These pictures show you what can happen to you if you don't take the messages in this book seriously. Don't think it won't happen to you as that is exactly what all the sufferers mentioned in this book thought. I will do everything I possibly can to make sure it won't happen to me though! Are you in with me? Sure hope so.

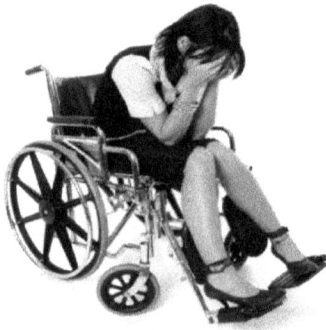

Do you want to end up like this by the age of 50? This is a very realistic outcome for children who start using modern electronic devices at the age of 8 and use them constantly every single day for many hours.

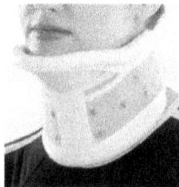

Or is this neck support collar what you want to be wearing when you are 40 because otherwise you have an unbearable pain in your neck because you've used your neck muscles in the wrong position for many years? Source: www.support4physio.com

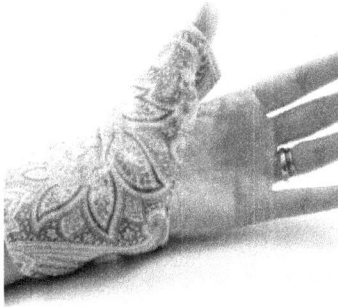

Source:www.theferriswheelshop.com

Or perhaps you want to wear a thumb wrap all the time for your texting thumb that hurts? They manufacturer these now in designs that are colourful and therefore appealing to youngsters. Surely that must tell you that texting thumb is a huge problem.

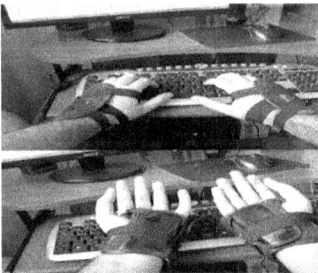

Or is this how you want to be typing when you're 30? Wearing gloves because without them you are simply in too much agony to type! Source: http://en.wikipedia.org/wiki/File:Luva.jpg

Chapter 3) Carpal Tunnel Syndrome - Treatment

The initial treatment for Carpal Tunnel Syndrome will be to take conservative measures. The patient will usually be advised to rest the affected hand and if it is determined that the symptoms have been caused by repetitive work such as typing or shop work, then the doctor might suggest that a wrist splint or hand splint is worn until the symptoms start to ease. Studies have indicated that wearing a carpal tunnel splint or a carpal tunnel wrist brace can be helpful in reducing symptoms when worn at night.

Dr Nathan Wei of the Arthritis Treatment Center outlines the treatments available for patients with CTS.

"Conservative management of Carpal Tunnel Syndrome consists of splinting, abstaining from activities that might have brought the problem on, physical therapy, exercises, massage, anti-inflammatory medicines, and steroid injection."

"Unfortunately, these don't always work in more serious or chronic cases."

a)Pain killers

In the early stages of Carpal Tunnel Syndrome, conservative measures will be the first course of action. This will include prescribing the patient painkillers to help them manage their discomfort and if the symptoms are chronic then the doctor might refer the patient to a pain clinic where the medical staff can advise the patient on the pain control methods that are available to them and suggest tools that can be useful for managing everyday tasks.

b) Anti-inflammatory Medication

If inflammation is thought to be contributing to the symptoms then an anti-inflammatory will be prescribed. These are usually given in the form of ibuprofen or naproxen. However, these types of drugs – which are commonly known as non-steroidal anti-inflammatory drugs – can cause stomach problems such as bleeding if they are taken regularly so they should not be taken in the long-term.

Muscle relaxants and nonsteroidal anti-inflammatory drugs (NSAIDs) such as Naproxen and Ibufrofen reduce pain and swelling.

c) Steroids

There is some debate as to how beneficial anti-inflammatory medication is for patients with Carpal Tunnel Syndrome, however, it is still often prescribed and if inflammation is present then this type of medication can help reduce the swelling, which can contribute to the symptoms of CTS.

However, some experts are of the opinion that steroids are a better option for treating the symptoms of CTS.

Corticosteroid is injected into soft tissue for short-term pain relief. Steroid injections can have negative side effects and should be considered carefully.

d) Rest

Patients will be told to avoid the activity that has caused or contributed to their condition if they can. For some people, this might not be possible, especially if they are in a manual job that involves using the hands and wrists a lot. In this case, adaptations will have to be made to the workstation or the employer will have to consider putting the employee on different duties until they are able to resume their normal role.

e) Ice

Ice can be useful in controlling swelling and easing pain, but should only be used for short periods of time and not directly against the skin. Patients with a lack of feeling in their hands or wrists should take care when using ice as they might not feel the ice if it begins to burn the skin.

f) Occupational Therapists

An occupational therapist is vital for helping patients with conditions such as Carpal Tunnel Syndrome to stay in work. They can offer advice on setting up the workstation so that the work environment is ergonomically sound, thus avoiding excessive stress on the upper body.

An occupational therapist can also give advice on other tools that will be suitable for managing the workload in other occupations such as jobs that require the use of hand tools or hairdressing, for example.

g) Exercise

Exercises for Carpal Tunnel Syndrome might also be suggested in order to maintain dexterity and strength. These exercises will often concentrate on stretching and strengthening the wrist area, however, as a weakening in the wrist from Carpal Tunnel Syndrome can often lead to the shoulders, forearms and biceps having to work much harder to compensate for the weakening in the wrist, strengthening these muscles is a good idea too.

h) Splints

A splint is a device used for support or immobilization of the spine or other limbs. Splints are often suggested to give the wrist some additional support. As well as providing support to the painful wrist, splints can also be a good way to prevent Carpal Tunnel Syndrome and the splints will hold the wrist in a neutral position when a person is typing or completing other repetitive actions, which will prevent an excessive strain being caused to the wrist area.

Diagnosis by a medical professional should guide treatment. Diagnosis explains the symptoms and opens up different treatment options. The effectiveness of the different treatments varies with the individual and with the type of CTS. The most common treatment options are as follows:

i) Physiotherapy

Light, infrared and ultraviolet rays, heat, electric current, massage, manipulation, and exercise.

k) Extended Scope Physiotherapy (ESP)

ESP practitioners study beyond the requirements of regular physiotherapists. They can request investigations such as nerve conduction scans and assist in diagnosis and treatment, listing for surgery, and referrals to other medical professionals.

l) Medication

As we have seen, Mmuscle relaxants and nonsteroidal anti-inflammatory drugs (NSAIDs) such as naproxen and ibuprofen reduce pain and swelling.

m) Immobilization

Lessens pain by immobilizing hands and arms with wrist braces, splints or elastic wrist supports. Often used at night with carpal tunnel syndrome. If overused, splints et al can do more damage than good, so should only be used on medical order.

n) Hypnosis

Pain management and healing in which patients visualize images that promote healing.

o) Heat packs

Heat packs can relieve chronic pain and relax muscles. May be used in combination with cold packs.

p) Chiropractic and osteopathic manipulation

Manipulate joints and muscles to restore them to normal positions and relieve tension.

q) Deep tissue massage

Relieves severe tension in the muscle connective tissue (called the fascia), focusing on the tissue below the surface muscles.

r) Trigger point massage/therapy

Releases painful trigger points (or muscle knots) that are the source of referred pain. Trigger points are tiny points in the muscle that are tender when touched.

s) Ultrasound therapy

High-intensity ultrasound can reduce pain and improve the healing of carpal tunnel syndrome and tendonitis. Ultrasound can also be used to aid the placement of cortisone injections.

t) Physical therapy

Stretching and strengthening exercises to reduce stress and recondition the body. This may also include postural retraining, ultrasound, heat and ice packs, or deep tissue massage.

u) Tiger Balm

Tiger Balm is wrapped on the painful areas and can give temporary relief.

Chapter 4) Carpal tunnel syndrome - Surgery

Carpal Tunnel Syndrome surgery may be recommended if symptoms last for a period of six months or longer. Physicians may also recommend RSI surgery for other advanced conditions. Surgery for RSIs are not always effective (the failure rate is over 50 percent) and is usually considered as a last resort.

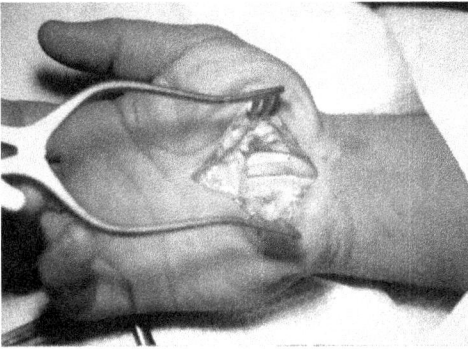

Carpal Tunnel Surgery Source:
http://commons.wikimedia.org/wiki/File:Carpal_Tunnel_Syndrom e,_Operation.jpg

If the symptoms are severe and conservative treatments have been unsuccessful, it will be time to start thinking about surgery. Surgery will only normally be considered when the symptoms have persisted for six months or more.

As the rehabilitation process for wrist surgery can be a lengthy one for some people –and as there is a chance that the symptoms can reoccur after surgery – the patient needs to find out all they can about the operation, the recovery time and the possible complications.

1) Open Release Surgery

During the surgery, the surgeon will make a cut through the carpal tendon. This will act to release the compression on the median nerve. It is quite a simple procedure and it is carried out under a local anaesthetic. This type of surgery is known as open release surgery and would normally be carried out under a day case basis unless there are other medical issues to be taken into consideration.

2) Endoscopic Carpal Tunnel Surgery

Endoscopic Carpal Tunnel release surgery or keyhole surgery is another option when it comes to carpal tunnel release surgery. This surgical option might be preferred by many patients as there is less pain post-surgery. During the operation two small incisions will be made. A camera will be inserted so that the surgeon can view the tissues on the screen. The surgeon will then make an incision into the carpal (wrist) tendon.

As with the open release procedure, keyhole surgery will be carried out under a local anaesthetic and there should be no need for a hospital stay unless there is an underlying medical condition to take into consideration.

Your surgeon will advise you to keep your hand moving in order to limit the amount of swelling and maintain dexterity.

After the carpal tunnel release surgery, patients will often be advised to wear a wrist brace or carpal tunnel brace after the surgery to help aid healing.

As with all types of surgery, there will be some risks. In the case of carpal tunnel surgery, patients could develop an infection at the site of the operation. To avoid this, antibiotics might be prescribed ahead of the operation.

There is also a chance that the nerves or tendons could be damaged during the procedure. Some patients might also go on to develop pain at the site of the scar and there may be a loss of muscle strength due to the cutting of the carpal ligament.

3) Ultra-sound Guided Needle Release

This type of surgery might be less well-known; however a study by Nathan Wei M.D, Thomas B. Clark, D.C, RVT, and Daniel G. Malone, M.D has shown that ultra sound guided needle release could be a good alternative for patients with Carpal Tunnel Syndrome.

The surgery is much easier to perform and uses standard injection equipment along with ultrasound equipment. Many of the patients undergoing ultra-sound guided needle release said that they didn't experience any real pain during the surgery, except at the time when the anaesthetic was given; there was some minor discomfort in the days after the operation.

Following surgery, many of the patients involved in the trial reported getting relief from their symptoms. The doctors concluded that this type of surgery provided a viable alternative to the open release surgery that is commonly performed to reduce Carpal Tunnel symptoms.

This type of surgery is minimally invasive and the recovery time is quicker than with other forms of surgery.

Sufferer's story: *"I was rinsing off some spaghetti the other night and my fingers in the affected hand just let go of the colander - and the spaghetti landed in the sink. That was the end of another meal! I can't cut up my food properly or clean my teeth very well (although I have now bought a sonic wave toothbrush, which helps with this task). When the pain and motor function is really bad, it's embarrassing to have to ask someone to unzip/unbutton my jeans or trousers so I can go to the loo, or having to ask my husband to cut up my food for me because I can't manage to do this simple task myself."* Source: Watson, M. 2009. Investigating the experiences of people with RSI. http://etheses.qmu.ac.uk/

4) Carpal Tunnel Surgery- Recovery

After the Carpal Tunnel surgery the patient is likely to need around eight weeks to recover. However, healing times will vary according to many factors such as the age of the patient and any underlying medical conditions; recovery from Carpal Tunnel Syndrome can be a long, frustrating process for some.

Another factor that will contribute to the length of healing time involved will be the type of surgery used. If the surgery used was minimally invasive, then the recovery time is likely to be much quicker.

The surgeon is likely to advise that the patient begins to get back into activities gradually and doesn't do anything that will inhibit healing, cause pain or swelling, or cause a reoccurrence of the symptoms.

It is likely that the patient will be referred to a physiotherapist in order to get some exercises to improve dexterity, grip and overall hand strength. The patient might also be offered advice on how to avoid the symptoms of Carpal Tunnel Syndrome in the future.

Everyday activities such as car driving might be difficult post-surgery and patients should take their doctor's advice when it comes to returning to the activities they used to participate in.

Some patients might find that they are unable to continue in their line of work or find their usual work tasks difficult following surgery. If this is the case then the patient should ask to see an Occupational Therapist or ask if it is possible to have a change of duties at work. In addition, employers are required to make adjustments should an employee be suffering from an illness or injury that restricts them from completing their normal duties at work; this could include work place adaptations. For example, a patient recovering from this type of surgery might need to use a different desk, keyboard or mouse. In these circumstances, there are grants available to cover the cost of paying for new equipment, so it need not cost the employer anything.

In addition, if the patient is self-employed and needs similar adaptations to their work station to enable them to continue working, grants are available for them too.

In some cases, patients will also be referred to an occupational therapist. An occupational therapist will work with a patient to address any postural issues or poor work place ergonomics that could have contributed to the development of the symptoms.

They will also offer advice on returning to work and on using tools to make the work and home environment more ergonomically friendly.

Chapter 5) Carpal Tunnel Syndrome - A Natural Approach

Many people don't like the thought of medication and prefer to use more natural treatments to help manage their symptoms. This book does not advocate one form of treatment over another, however, it is certainly worthwhile to highlight some of the natural ways of coping with Carpal Tunnel Syndrome.

Vitamins and natural remedies are only ever meant to compliment treatment, and not to replace conventional medicine and this should be borne in mind when deciding whether or not to try more natural supplements.

The following chapter will detail vitamins, herbs and natural treatments that patients with Carpal Tunnel Syndrome say have brought them some relief from their carpal tunnel symptoms.

There is one firm guideline to consider before supplementing the diet with vitamins, minerals, herbal remedies or any form of alternative therapy and that is to speak to your GP or consultant first so they can discuss with you whether they think it is worthwhile adding extra supplements to the diet or not.

Speaking to your medical team is imperative if you are on any other medication as some nutritional and herbal supplements can have contraindications with medication. Some of these are included in the precautions section under each vitamin, however, this list of possible contraindications is not exhaustive so speak to your medical team before supplementing your diet.

If you are scheduled for surgery, you will also need to advise the medical team if you have been taking any supplements/herbal remedies.

Some vitamins have shown promise in the treatment of Carpal Tunnel Syndrome. However, there are still some mixed opinions about whether this is an effective treatment for patients as various studies have shown mixed results.

This chapter will detail some of the supplements that are believed to help reduce the symptoms in some patients. As everyone is different, not everyone will benefit from them, but they may well bring relief to some patients with Carpal Tunnel Syndrome..

Patients should speak to a doctor before beginning any new nutritional regimen in order to prevent the possibility of any drug interactions.

Also detailed in this chapter are details of foods that are naturally high in the suggested vitamins and rather than supplementing the diet with extra vitamins, many experts suggest getting the vitamins the body needs from the diet itself.

It would also be a good idea to get some tests carried out to see if you are deficient in any of these vitamins as sometimes the symptoms only desist because a patient lacks a certain vitamin and supplementing the diet has corrected the lack of that particular nutrient.

When supplementing with B vitamins, it is a good idea to take a B complex supplement as well to avoid a depletion of any of the other B vitamins in the body.

1) Tingling and Numbness

For many people the discomfort caused by the tingling sensation experienced by people with Carpal Tunnel Syndrome can be among the most distressing.

B vitamins have been shown to be effective for some patients experiencing these symptoms and some experts believe that Carpal Tunnel Syndrome can result due to a lack of vitamin B6.

a) Vitamin B6

Patients taking vitamin B6 to help control their symptoms report a reduction in pain, while other studies have shown that symptoms such as numbness and tingling in the affected fingers were not reduced.

Other studies suggest that B6 can help a patient to avoid surgery – or at least delay it. In the trials carried out, B6 was given as a 200mg dose, however, it is important that a patient does not self-medicate as B6 taken in high doses can cause nerve problems in itself; patients have been known to develop neuropathy, which leads to symptoms such as pain, tingling, numbness and problems walking when taking high doses of vitamin B6.

Dietary Sources:

B6 can be obtained from green vegetables, pulses, potatoes, grains and breakfast cereals.

Contraindications

B6 should not be taken by patients on certain medications. This includes patients on medication for arthritis, TB, blood pressure and asthma.

It is also advisable not to take B6 supplements if you are on some form of anti-depressant drugs, antibiotics, chemotherapy drugs and drugs for Parkinson's disease.

Diabetics might find that their blood sugars are affected when taking B6.

b) Vitamin B12

Vitamin B12 has been shown to reduce pain in patients with Carpal Tunnel Syndrome. A deficiency of B12 can also cause symptoms such as tingling and numbness as a lack of B12 can contribute to the development of neuropathy and can be common in vegetarians.

Before supplementing with B12, speak to your doctor or consultant about the possibility of getting some blood tests completed to see if your B12 levels are normal as if you are deficient in this essential vitamin, correcting the deficiency could help to reduce numbness, tingling and some of the strange sensations that often occur as the result of nerve damage.

In one study carried out in Japan, patients were given vitamin B12 in the form of mecobalamin. Patients participating in the study experienced an improvement in the sensory symptoms of Carpal Tunnel Syndrome.

The study also found that this form was safe to take and didn't cause any noticeable side effects. The vitamin was given in the form of an oral supplement.

Vitamin B12 is also available in the form of Methylcobalamin. This form of B12 is believed to be much better absorbed than other forms of B12 supplements and they are easier to digest.

These tablets can be taken every 2-3 days and can help reduce symptoms such as tingling and numbness in some patients. However, this may just be due to an underlying deficiency of B12 that might have been contributing to the symptoms. B12 is essential for the neurological system and for nerve function, which is why patients that lack this vitamin can begin to develop symptoms of neuropathy.

Dietary Sources:

B12 is readily available in fortified breakfast cereals, grains, red meat and fish. Dairy products also contain B12.

Precautions:

Patients on medications such as antibiotics and medication to control acid reflux or ulcers should not supplement with vitamin B12 without consulting their doctor.

c) Vitamin B2

Studies have also suggested that B2 might be beneficial for patients with Carpal Tunnel Syndrome. B2 – or riboflavin – is important for keeping the nerves healthy and a severe lack of this vitamin can lead to symptoms such as muscle weakness and problems with co-ordination.

Dietary Sources:

Cereals and breads contain vitamin B2. The vitamin can also be added to the diet by including meat, cheese and bananas.

Precautions:

Anti-depressants, Luminal and Benemid are just some of the drugs that can interact with riboflavin.

d) Alpha Lipoic Acid

A study has shown that Alpha Lipoic Acid, when taken in conjunction with gamma-linoleic acid, helped to improve symptoms. Electromyography results were also improved.

The study concluded that this combination is best taken in the early stages of Carpal Tunnel Syndrome.

Alpha Lipoic acid was given as 60omg dose and GLA was given as a 300mg dosage.

Precautions:

Alpha lipoic acid might interfere with thyroid medication.

e) Magnesium

Magnesium is an essential mineral that is known to relax the muscles and calm muscle spasms. The mineral is also vital to the health of the nervous system and aids the healthy transmission of impulses.

Some experts argue that a lack of magnesium can contribute to CTS; a lack of magnesium can cause numbness, tingling and cramps.

It can be taken in tablet form and it is best taken as a supplement that contains calcium and boron.

Magnesium can also be bought as a spray and some patients with Carpal Tunnel Syndrome report a reduction in the tingling sensations they experience after they have massaged in some magnesium oil.

Dietary Sources

Nuts, pulses, green vegetables, yogurt and soya all contain magnesium.

Precautions:

Magnesium can interact with diuretics, antibiotics and medicines that are used to treat osteoporosis. The mineral can also interact with PPI medications, so advice should be taken before using supplements.

2) Natural Approaches to Inflammation

Often, Carpal Tunnel Syndrome is the result of inflammation in the tendons. The swelling that occurs due the inflammation can lead to the median nerve becoming entrapped.

However, if you are already taking prescribed anti-inflammatories, the following suggested remedies should not be taken alongside them.

a) Evening Primrose Oil

If inflammation has contributed to the development of Carpal Tunnel Syndrome, then supplementing with evening primrose oil can be beneficial. It's the GLA or gamma linoleic acid that is the active ingredient in evening primrose oil.

GLA can also be obtained from blackcurrant or borage oils and spirulina is also an excellent source of GLA.

Precautions:

Evening Primrose Oil should not be taken by people on blood thinning drugs or anti-coagulant drugs; people on immuno suppressants should also avoid supplementing their diet with evening primrose oil.

b) Fish Oil

As well as being beneficial for maintaining a healthy heart and good circulation, fish oil is also helpful for reducing inflammation. While more research needs to be done into this area, initial research has shown that patients with Carpal Tunnel Syndrome reported a reduction in their pain levels when taking fish oil. Fish oil can also be beneficial to patients suffering from other types of neurological pain.

Fish oil can be taken in capsule form or in liquid form.

Dietary Sources

Omega 3, the active ingredient in fish oil, can be obtained from nuts, seeds, omega eggs, vegetable oils and fish.

Precautions:

People on blood thinning or anti-coagulant medication should not supplement their diet with fish oil and should speak to their medical team before adding extra omega 3 rich foods to their diet.

c) MSM

This sulphur rich supplement reduces inflammation, which in turn can help to ease swelling, thus limiting the pressure put on the nerves.

It can also help to reduce muscle spasm, which can also contribute to the pain and discomfort in patients with Carpal Tunnel Syndrome.

MSM is not an effective treatment for everyone, and it needs to be taken for a long time before patients can expect to see a reduction in their symptoms.

This supplement is often used by arthritis patients to help manage pain levels and maintain mobility.

MSM is available in capsule form.

Dietary Sources:

Foods that contain MSM include fruits, vegetables and grains, however, to get a significant amount into the diet, it is better to use supplements.

Precautions:

More research needs to be done before it can be established if there are any contraindications with medications. Anyone considering taking this supplement should seek medical advice to check it will not have a negative effect on any prescribed medications that they are on.

Pregnant women or women who are breastfeeding should also seek expert advice.

d) Bromelian

Bromelian is the natural enzyme that comes from pineapple. Bromelian is believed to have many health benefits and it is often used as a natural way to reduce inflammation and swelling.

If surgery is deemed necessary, bromelian can be used to help reduce some of the post-operative inflammation.

This supplement can be brought in tablet form.

Dietary Sources:

Pineapple

Precautions:

Bromelian can cause excess bleeding in some individuals so it shouldn't be taken by patients on blood thinning or anti-coagulant drugs.

Bromelian should also be avoided by patients on sedatives or drugs for depression.

e) Vitamin C

Vitamin C can be helpful to control inflammation. It is also beneficial to patients with tendon problems as it helps with the production of collagen.

Vitamin C will also help to heal any bruising that might result due to surgery and it can speed up healing time; the vitamin plays an important role in the health of the vessels.

Vitamin C is available in effervescent form, capsules, powders and tablets. For best results, find a supplement that has added bioflavonoids and make sure that it doesn't have added sugar.

Dietary Sources:

Fruits and vegetables are among the best sources for adding vitamin C to the diet.

Precautions:

Diabetics might find that vitamin C will affect their blood sugar levels. Patients with anaemia should also be careful when taking vitamin C, because it is known to increase the absorption of iron.

f) Ginger

Some people find ginger an effective home remedy for Carpal Tunnel Syndrome. Ginger is known for its anti-inflammatory effects so if inflammation is contributing to the pain levels, then this herb might be beneficial. Ginger also acts to warm the affected area and will help to boost and improve circulation.

Ginger can be added to the diet as a supplement or added to the diet in powder form.

Ginger muscle rubs are also available and these will help to warm the muscles and help reduce muscle fatigue.

Another way of using ginger is by using it as an essential oil. To apply to the painful area, add a few drops to a base oil such as sweet almond oil and massage into the skin.

Precautions:

Ginger should not be taken by people who are on blood thinning medication and people with gall stones should seek advice before supplementing with ginger.

If using a lotion or essential oil, then take care when applying to sensitive or delicate skin.

g) Circumin
This spice has a number of medicinal uses, and can help to reduce inflammation and pain. It can also help to encourage the healing process and is useful for those suffering from a sports injury such as tendonitis.

h) Boswellia
Boswellia is another natural anti-inflammatory. It can help to sooth pain and can be taken as a supplement or used as a cream to reduce pain and swelling.

Boswellia or Frankincense also works has an analgesic and can help to provide pain relief in nerve problems.

The cream is easy to apply to the affected area and will be absorbed quickly.

i) Pycnogenol
Pycnogenol acts as a powerful anti-oxidant and it is thought to have many health benefits. For instance, patients with diabetes

might find this supplement, which is an extract of pine bark, effective as it is believed to help with retinopathy, a complication of long-term diabetes that occurs in some patients.

However, Pycnogenol also has strong anti-inflammatory properties and could be helpful in the healing process.

Pycnogenol should not be taken by patients on corticosteroid drugs or immunosuppressant's.

j) Green Tea

Green tea contains high levels of anti-oxidants. It is thought to lower blood sugar levels, reduce blood pressure, protect the body from cancer and lower cholesterol levels.

In addition, it works as an anti-inflammatory, which could help limit pain and swelling.

While many of the green tea products available contain caffeine, there are now some caffeine free products available if they are preferred and there are also some flavoured versions for those that don't like the strong taste of the tea.

It can also be served with honey to add some natural sweetness to it.

3) Lotions and Cream

As well as the products detailed below, there are many other products on the market that patients might find helpful. Massage creams come in many different forms and it is just a matter of finding one that suits your needs. For instance, if your hands feel very hot, look for one that has a cooling effect or look for one of the neuropathy lotions that has been designed to reduce the uncomfortable symptoms associated with nerve entrapment.

a) Arnica

Arnica is a homeopathic remedy often used for sprains and strains. However, it can be helpful for patients who have undergone surgery as it will help to reduce the swelling and bruising that might occur afterwards.

In addition, arnica has been found to be effective in reducing pain following carpal tunnel release surgery. A study was conducted among 37 patients who had undergone bilateral endoscopic carpal-tunnel release surgery.

The patients in the trial were given arnica in the form of tablets and cream and they reported a significant reduction in pain when compared with the placebo group.

b) CT Cream

This cream has been developed for patients with Carpal Tunnel Syndrome and repetitive strain injuries. It can also be used by patients with tennis elbow, arthritis or other inflammations.

The cream contains all natural ingredients and many patients report a reduction in their symptoms after using this cream.

c) EMLA Cream

EMLA cream contains lidocaine and prilocaine as its active ingredients. It acts as a topical anaesthesia and studies have shown that patients using the cream have reported a reduction in their pain levels; the majority of the patients using the cream didn't experience any side effects.

The cream is readily available online without prescription, but should not be used by patients on other medications or with an underlying condition.

d) Other Creams

Penetrex cream and Topricin creams are also natural products that have been developed for patients with CTS.

Penetrex Cream is a topical pain reliever and contains only natural ingredients. The cream can be used up to four times a day and it is useful to apply it when having a massage of the affected area. It is also a good idea to use it last thing at night as this is often when the pain is at its worse.

Topricin Cream comes in several varieties and it is safe for diabetics. There is also a foot cream for patients with neuropathy and experiencing pain in their feet.

The cream is available on Amazon or from other online retailers. If there are any problems obtaining the cream then it can be bought direct from the manufacturer's website for customers in the US.

Chapter 6) Alternative Therapies for Carpal Tunnel Syndrome

For patients keen to avoid undergoing surgery for Carpal Tunnel Syndrome, alternative therapies can be a good option to explore. Patients will often experience mixed results, and what works well for one patient might not work for another.

Finding natural therapists in your area is easy and there are many directories online that will list therapists that practice locally; before trying any form of alternative remedies, however, speak to your doctor first. Listed in this chapter are some therapies that have shown to be beneficial to patients with Carpal Tunnel Syndrome.

1) Acupuncture

Some patients find acupuncture an effective treatment for Carpal Tunnel Syndrome. Treatments such as acupuncture are sometimes available on the NHS so if you are a patient in the UK then it is a good idea to ask if acupuncture treatments are available in your area.

If you are undergoing treatment at a pain clinic, the specialist there can often refer a patient to services such as acupuncture, which are offered by the local hospital. However, waiting lists are long, and if the pain is severe and the patient is keen for relief, then paying to go to see a therapist privately is the best option. Prices start from £35-40 a session, and depending on the severity of the symptoms, up to ten sessions might be required.

Many patients find relief from their pain through acupuncture and it can be a helpful way to reduce muscle spasms; one study has demonstrated that acupuncture can be as beneficial as taking steroid medication for some patients.

It is best for patients with only mild to moderate symptoms of Carpal Tunnel Syndrome and there are no noticeable side effects with patients undergoing acupuncture for Carpal Tunnel Syndrome.

2) Osteopathy

Osteopathy can be a valuable tool for treating and diagnosing Carpal Tunnel Syndrome. An osteopath might also be able to identify where the entrapment is.

Osteopaths believe in treating the whole of the body, and not just the affected area. An osteopath will use gentle manipulation techniques and massage to help relieve the symptoms of Carpal Tunnel Syndrome.

3) Trigger Point Therapy

Trigger point therapy involves finding the trigger point of the pain as pain can often be referred from somewhere else. For instance, a person with earache or frequent headaches might have a problem with their jaw, or patients with problems in their shoulder might have pain in their lower arm/wrist, or vice versa.

When these trigger points are identified, pressing on them will send pain to another area of the body, thus allowing the therapist to identify the trigger point that is causing or contributing to the pain.

Osteopaths will often use trigger point therapy in their treatments and books about this form of therapy are available for patients who want to find out more.

However, in some patients, pressing a trigger point can make the pain worse, and there is no way of telling if the patient is going to be one of those people who find a worsening of their symptoms until they have tried this form of therapy.

4) Acupressure

In many ways, acupressure is similar to acupuncture. Practitioners of acupressure believe that by asserting gentle force on various pressure points throughout the body, it can help to relieve symptoms elsewhere in the body. Many people find that this is a helpful form of pain relief and claim that they feel they have more energy afterwards.

5) Yoga

Some key yoga exercises were featured in chapter two, however, yoga in general can be extremely beneficial for patients with CTS. First of all, it can help improve posture and as there is often a postural element to Carpal Tunnel Syndrome, yoga can be helpful in reducing or preventing the symptoms of this nerve entrapment.

Yoga is also a highly effective means of relaxing and reducing tension throughout the entire body, and not just the wrist area. As many CTS sufferers will have developed their condition due to overuse, it is also likely that they will have areas of accumulated tension throughout their body and yoga can alleviate this.

For anyone working in a highly repetitive task, yoga could go a long way in helping to dissolve tension and reduce aches and pains all over the body.

When practicing yoga, focus on the wrists, shoulders, hands, fingers and forearms. The upper back area will also require some attention as well, especially for patients who work in front of computers.

Follow each yoga session with a deep relaxation session or a guided meditation to focus on areas that are tight and tense. Yoga is best practiced early in the evening, or if there isn't time, a short session before bed that focuses on key areas, along with a deep relaxation, will be enough to start underdoing some of the tight, tense muscles.

6) Massage

Massage is an effective means of reducing tightness, tension and pain in the muscles. If your occupation involves a lot of repetitive work, then you are one of the people that can really benefit from a regular massage session, even if you aren't feeling any discomfort.

The pain from repetitive strain injuries such as Carpal Tunnel Syndrome rarely comes out of nowhere and it can often be due an accumulation of repetitive actions. Although overusing the muscles/tendons might not show any symptoms to begin with, over time they often will.

Use a regular massage session to prevent the muscles and tendons from becoming too tight and to prevent the onset of pain from setting in.

7) Alexander Technique

If posture has played a part in the development of your CTS symptoms then using therapies that can help re-educate your body and train your posture to help reduce to pain.

8) Pilates

Pilates is another excellent way to improve posture and reduce pain when you move.

Pilates use small, controlled movements that help to strengthen the core muscles of the body and improve the way you sit, stand and walk.

9) Chiropractor

A Chiropractor can help a patient with Carpal Tunnel Syndrome by manipulating the soft tissue of the affected wrist. A chiropractor might also choose to focus on other areas of the upper body in order to reduce the symptoms of CTS.

Sufferer's story: *"I'm a 17 year old male. I have been having some joint pain in the last few weeks. Very recently, I noticed that my fingers were getting stiff. It started from the little finger in my left hand which was really stiff. When I bring any movements to the finger, it moves in a really edgy or a jerky way instead of the usual, smooth movements. I sit in front of the computer for really long hours and I felt that this was the reason for it. So I started taking frequent breaks but I don't think it helped that much. This problem has been getting worse from day to day. Yesterday I noticed the same thing happen in my right hand too. The little finger in both hands does not have limited range but movement (jerky). And this same problem is spreading to the other fingers as well. No swelling has been observed but lack of movement, mild (sometimes severe in mornings) pain, loss of grip and mild pain on wrist are noticeable. Symptoms are worse at times after I wake up from sleep where a huge portion of my fingers are stiff and I experience difficultly getting a strong grip. The problems are also worse on colder days. Source: chatastrophy on Medhelp.org 10 August 2008 (Capitalization and punctuation added for ease of reading.)*

10) Biofeedback

Measures stresses and offers methods for relaxing mind and muscles.

11) Cognitive Behavioural Therapy (CBT)

Approach to controlling and managing pain and depression.

12) Tai Chi

Improves posture with moving meditation/martial art. It strengthens muscles, improves flexibility and stimulates healing.

13) Bowen Technique

Promotes rebalancing and proper alignment. RSI-sufferers who find most touch painful may like the very gentle touch of the Bowen Technique.

14) Feldenkrais Method

Improves body awareness through bodywork and gentle exercise. Retrains the body, making all movements smooth and efficient.

15) Shiatsu

Japanese finger pressure therapy targets acupuncture points.

16) Reflexology

Removes blockages in nerve endings, allowing nerves to function better.

17) Craniosacral Therapy

Removes restrictions in cerebrospinal fluid and energy flow in the body.

18) Magnet Therapy

Increases circulation, which helps the healing process.

19) Relaxation Techniques

Reduces physical and mental stress, tension, and pain.

The Mind Body Prescription is a book by Dr. John E. Sarno about pain syndromes such as RSI. Some people say if they understand the pain, they can deal with it better.

20) Walking or moving

Listed last but certainly not the least important: you will be surprised how much good walking can do for your body. Get yourself to a park or just go for a walk outside your house.

Chapter 7) Coping with Carpal Tunnel Syndrome

Simple coping strategies can make life so much easier. The overall coping strategy is to be aware of what works for you and what doesn't, take breaks before you hurt, and use your body gently.

For additional practical tips, go to JAN (the Job Accommodation Network); this website has a searchable database of ideas and accommodations, at https://askjan.org/media/cumu.htm. The Vendors list at the end of this book includes companies that sell devices for daily living.

1) Shopping

- Buy groceries and supplies in smaller quantities so you don't have to do as much lifting and carrying.

- Make more trips instead of carrying too many bags at once.

- Shop at stores that deliver.

- Avoid shoulder bags for carrying. Use rucksacks that have two straps and a waistband for distributing your weight. Or use wheeled carry bags.

- If you have to carry a bag, try resting the handle over your forearm instead of gripping the handle with your fingers. The muscles in the arm are bigger and stronger than those in your fingers, so they can do more work without injury.

2) Out in the World

- Shaking hands poses a dilemma for CTS-sufferers. A handshake can be painful for sore hands, but if the other person is a business associate or new acquaintance, you may not want them to know you can't shake hands and you don't want to seem rude. Here are ideas to solve the problem: you can gently put your hands around the other person's forearm, bow slightly, or hold a light object in your hand so it's obvious you can't shake. Your objective is to protect your hand without appearing discourteous.

- Instead of clapping, shout "bravo!" Or, stamp your feet, tap your palm with a program, or pretend to clap without actually touching your hands together. Or, try the applause used by deaf audiences: raise your hands, stretch out your fingers, and twist your wrists.

- If you take public transportation, avoid rush hour if you can so you can be sure of getting a seat. If you don't get a seat, put your bag between your feet instead of holding it; loop your arm around a pole instead of trying to hold on with your hands.

- Driving—don't do it unless you have complete control over your vehicle. Power steering; automatic transmission; and power windows, mirrors, locks and seats make it easier.

- Use an easy reach seatbelt handle to reach your seatbelt without straining.

- Use feet and legs instead of hands to open and close doors. Push doors open with your hip, foot, or shoulder. As much as possible, let other people open doors for you.

- Push doorbells and elevator buttons with an elbow, knuckle, or umbrella.

3) Communicating

- It's easy to become isolated by the pain and limitations of RSIs, so it's important to keep lines of communication open. Your familiar ways of communicating may become uncomfortable. Here are ideas for keeping in touch.

- Call people on the phone instead of sending emails or texts.

- Use handsets and speakerphones when talking on the telephone.

- Easy-touch keyboards take less hand effort.

- Use the auto-dial feature on the telephone, or get a voice-activated phone.

- For writing, choose pens that have thick, soft grips and write with very little pressure, like old-fashioned fountain pens. If you can't find thick enough pens, wrap bubble wrap or a foam hair curler around a pen.

- STOP TEXTING AND START TALKING.

The following ideas are adapted from hints from members of Australia's RSI Association:

4) Dressing and Grooming

- Buy clothing with zippers instead of buttons and shoes that slip on or have Velcro closures instead of laces.

- Buy skirts and slacks with elastic waists.

- Avoid clothing that needs to be ironed. You can reduce wrinkles by hanging up clothes after you wear them or wash them, putting clothes in the dryer, or hanging them near the shower so steam can release wrinkles.

- Use a shoehorn. A shoe and boot valet lets you put on and take off shoes with one hand without bending down.

- Use a reaching tool to access, for example, socks on the floor or jumpers on high shelves.

- Store clothes on shelves instead of in bureau drawers.

- Zipper pulls, long handle hairbrushes, button pulls, and bra aids make grooming and dressing easier.

- Use one-handed nail clippers to keep nails trim; long fingernails interfere with good typing technique.

-       Hang your head down when brushing or blow drying so you don't have to raise your arms up.

-       Repair hems, seams, and tears with fabric glue instead of needle and thread.

5) Around the House

-       Use kitchen equipment with thicker, easier to grip handles. Wrap foam hair curlers, bubble wrap, or foam handles around pencils, pens, and eating utensils to make them easier to hold onto. OXO Good Grips (www.oxo.com) is a line of kitchen tools and dining utensils with soft, thick grips.

-       Use bendable dining utensils for easier holding and cutting.

-       Use double-handed mugs, which are easier to lift and hold on to.

-       Use a bookstand so you don't have to hold the book in your hands.

-       Use very sharp, serrated knives for dining and preparing food. They take less effort.

-       Fit lamp switch enlargers over existing light switches to make them easier to grasp and turn.

-       Use automatic staplers and spring-loaded scissors.

-       Go electrical: can opener, knife sharpener, knives, card shuffler, razor, etc.

-       Cover keys with key holders to make them easier to grip.

-        Store frequently used items on shelves at waist level so you don't have to reach overhead for them. Items you use daily should stay on the countertop.

-        Install door handle grips, turners, or extenders over round doorknobs. Turn the doorknob with finger, elbow, or closed fist. Available from Good Grips (http://www.greatgrips.com), Assistive Devices Key (http://www.assistivedeviceskey.com/) and Life with Ease http://www.lifewithease.com/

6) Gardening

Gardening has both physical and psychological benefits: it gets your body moving and soothes your mind. You may have to adopt new gardening methods and tools; fortunately adaptive gardening has many practical tips and new and accomplished gardeners.

-        Build raised bed gardens so you don't have to bend or reach so far. Thus, if you have mobility limitations you can still garden.

-        Reduce the size of your garden. Compact gardens can be amazingly beautiful…and less work.

-        Use a heavy mulch to reduce the amount of weeding, watering, and fertilizing you have to do.

-        Instead of digging or roto-tilling your vegetable garden use the no-till method.

-        Don't use power tools.

-        Lightweight hand tools, long-handled tools, and padded handles all make tools easier to use.

-        Pistol grips on hand tools and bent handles on digging tools help keep your hand in the neutral position and so need less force to use.

-        Install a watering system so you don't have to carry a hose or watering can. Better still grow plants that thrive in your location without much water. If you do turn on a hose now and then install plastic fittings (tap turners) that make it easier.

-        Avoid pruning by planting trees and shrubs that grow slowly and/or don't require annual trimming.

-        Use wheelbarrows or garden carts for carrying. Don't overload them. It's better to make more trips than to strain your arms, hands, and shoulders with heavy loads.

-        Never work to the point of pain. Pace yourself and take frequent breaks.

The American Horticultural Therapy Association (www.ahta.org), the Canadian Horticultural Therapy Association (www.chta.ca), and Trellis (www.trellisscotland.org.uk) focus on gardening for people with disabilities. As the American Horticultural Therapy Association website puts it: "The therapeutic benefits of peaceful garden environments have been understood since ancient times."

7) Managing Pain

CTS can be very painful. The pain itself can be debilitating but most CTS-sufferers learn to manage the pain. Pain management is partly physical and partly mental and a number of the treatment options listed here are self-care techniques that you can use to deal with your pain:

-        If it hurts when you do a certain activity, stop doing it but don't stop moving altogether. Moving keeps the blood circulating and speeds up recovery.

-        Cold is a quick and easy way to temporarily reduce inflammation and swelling, and therefore pain. Use it straight after you do something that causes pain and for up to 15 times a day. Apply ice or cold water directly on the painful spot, but keep the ice moving (don't let it sit on your skin) for about a minute. Let the spot where you applied the ice warm up before you start an activity. Important note: cold treatment is only recommended when inflammation occurs. Heat is better for general aches and pains when there is no inflammation.

-        Heat relaxes sore muscles and makes them easier to move. Use heat packs, warm water or hot water bottles for moist heat. You can buy microwavable heat packs, which a lot of people recommend.

-        Exercise relieves pain, speeds up healing, reduces stress, and decreases anxiety and depression. Try walking, swimming, yoga, or biking.

-        Many people find listening to music soothing.

-        Stretches and strengthening exercises relieve stress.

-        Self-massage relieves pain. You can massage one hand/arm with the other hand, roll a hard rubber ball (tennis or squash ball) between your arm and a table or between your back and the floor, use a massage machine, or use simple massage tools.

-        Professional massage relaxes muscles and reduces pain. The choice of massage is individual but many RSI sufferers prefer a light touch, although my mum simply loves deep tissue massage and always gets a lot of pain relief from it.

-        Herbal oils, menthol creams, and rubbing ointments can soothe sore muscles and bring relief.

-        Mind-body approaches to pain management use the power of thoughts and feelings to reduce pain and support healing. Biofeedback, meditation, and cognitive behaviour therapy (CBT) are three of many mind-body techniques that you can learn and practice on your own.

-        Pain clinics can help with a variety of pain management techniques.

8) Stretching and Exercising

Moving the body releases endorphins, which reduce pain. It also decreases tension and improves muscle strength. It gets blood flowing throughout the body, nourishing the tissues and aiding healing. Exercise improves overall wellbeing, relieves depression and makes the body less vulnerable to injury.

There are two parts to exercise: stretching and strengthening. The stretching exercises in different sections of this book are designed to relieve tension in the parts of the body you overuse when you text, type, or use other electronic devices. It only takes seconds to stretch, so you can do it many times a day. Stretch while you wait for the bus, in between phone calls, when you take breaks from computing, while a clerk rings you up—whenever you have a free moment. Stretching should start slow and easy, increasing with steady pressure and stopping just before the point of pain. No bouncing, jerking or quick movements. The simple stretches described in this book should not hurt; stop if they do and seek medical attention. If you have an RSI, your doctor may discourage certain stretches, especially if you are in the acute phase.

Important: do not stretch whilst it hurts. If the stretching becomes painful, it is time to stop as you could be causing more damage.

Strengthening exercises are also important for recovering from RSIs, but they are not as simple a matter as stretching. Exercise can cause RSIs or make them worse. That's why you should consult a medical professional before starting or continuing an exercise program if you have RSI symptoms. A physical or occupational therapist, osteopath or chiropractor can prescribe the best exercises for your condition and show you how to do them correctly. RSI-sufferers should exercise under medical guidance which is why this book does not include strengthening exercises.

Chapter 8) Carpal Tunnel Syndrome – Exercises

While exercise can go a long way towards reducing tightness in the wrist area and can help to build up lost muscle, there is a limit to how much exercises can aid the treatment of Carpal Tunnel Syndrome.

Exercises for Carpal Tunnel Syndrome will not reduce the other symptoms of CTS such as numbness, tingling or pain, it will, however, help to keep the muscles mobile and carrying out regular stretching can help reduce some of the stress and tension that accumulates when doing repetitive actions.

This chapter details exercises that are designed to stretch the hands, wrists and fingers and exercises to build strength in the muscles. Yoga has been shown to be an effective way to relieve some of the symptoms of Carpal Tunnel Syndrome; yoga exercises that will stretch out the wrist, arm and hand area are also included in this chapter.

However, people experiencing severe symptoms of Carpal Tunnel Syndrome should not attempt any of these exercises and should instead consult the person responsible for their care before attempting any of them.

If the symptoms are less severe, and still only in the minor stages, then it is still a good idea to seek some advice as these exercises might not be suitable for everyone. Moreover, patients with additional medical issues will also need to take extra care before proceeding with any of the exercises detailed.

If the patient feels any discomfort during any of the exercises or after the exercise, they should be discontinued to avoid making the pain any worse.

The yoga exercises detailed in this chapter are probably best avoided by patients with severe symptoms of Carpal Tunnel Syndrome. However, yoga exercises that will release tension in the upper body area can be beneficial for patients with this condition and they can help prevent the development of CTS, especially in people whose job involves a lot of repetitive activity or whose job requires them to be sat in one position for long periods at a time.

Before doing any of the exercises, make sure that your hands are warm and circle the wrists to get the blood flowing. Warm muscles are easier to stretch than cold ones and this can help avoid muscle pulls or strains.

1) Hand Stretches

a) Prayer Stretch

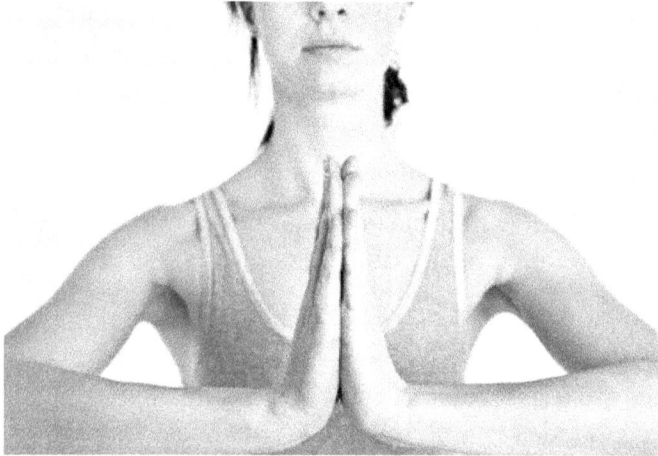

This simple stretch is ideal for gently relaxing the wrist area and releasing tightness from the muscles. It should be carried out regularly by people who do a lot of typing and get pain in their hands as a result.

Don't wait until the hands start to hurt before doing this exercise. Instead, practice it at regular intervals to help prevent tightness accumulating in the wrist area.

Directions:

To complete this stretch, simply hold the palms together in a prayer position. The stretch should be felt along the wrist. Hold the stretch for 5-30 seconds and repeat 3-5 times.

For those who want a gentler stretch there is another method of completing this stretch. Instead of holding the palms together, place one hand flat against the wall with the fingers pointing upwards, the same as they were in the previous stretch.

Hold the stretch until it can be felt along the wrist, but take care not to place too much pressure on the wrist when it is resting against the wall as this can create additional tension.

For another variation of the prayer stretch, a small ball can be placed between the hands. This will give a deeper, more intense stretch and should not be held for too long in case it causes pain or creates excess tension. Hold the stretch for 3-5 seconds to begin with and repeat the stretch three times; take a short break between each stretch. Once the wrist area loosens, this stretch will feel less intense and the exercise can be repeated more often.

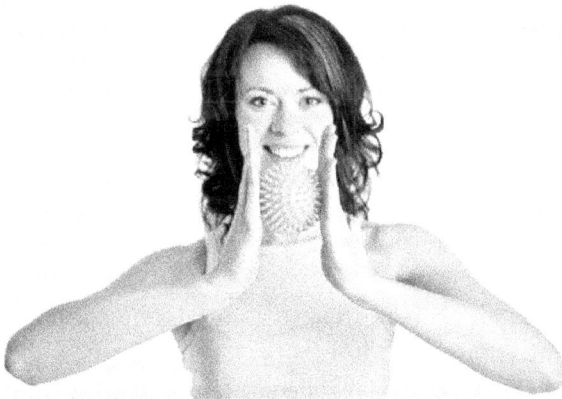

These stretches can be carried out at any point during the day and they are especially useful when you are carrying out work or participating in a hobby that requires a lot of repetitive motion.

As explained previously in the book, it is important not to wait until you get symptoms of pain before you do the exercises. Practicing the stretches can help to prevent the onset of pain and they are an excellent way of changing the action of the hands, thus helping to avoid repetitive strain.

The Handmaster Plus is an ideal size for assisting with this exercise and for keeping the palms an adequate distance apart for feeling the stretch.

b) Wrist Stretch

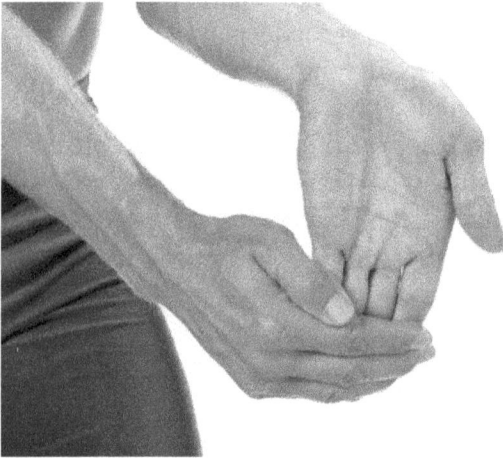

Once the wrist has been stretched in one direction, it is important to stretch the carpal out in the opposite direction in order to create a balanced stretch.

This stretch can be repeated 3-5 times. When fully extended, the wrist can be pulled gently to the left to feel the stretch on the inside of the wrist, or to the right to feel the stretch on the outside of the wrist. Only do this if the exercise can be done comfortably and don't try this if the tendons are over tight or if the joints are inflamed from arthritis.

In addition, this stretch can feel quite intense if the wrist area is not stretched out very often. If this is the case, just repeat the stretch once and repeat it as often as possible throughout the day. Taking the opportunity to do this stretch while waiting for a file to download or an application to start up is a good way of working this exercise into the daily routine. Practiced regularly, this exercise can go a long way to preventing the onset of wrist pain.

c) Wrist Rotating

Rotating the wrist is a good way to keep the wrist area relaxed and to avoid tension developing in the wrist. This is a good exercise to practice during the course of the day or when a lot of repetitive actions are being carried out. The exercise can also be used to gently warm the muscles before doing any of the wrist stretches in this chapter.

This exercise will also help to keep the muscles in the wrists from tightening up and will help to avoid stiffness in the wrist.

Directions:

Rotate the left wrist clockwise five times and then repeat the action counter clockwise. Make sure that the wrist is rotated as far as it will comfortably go, and make the circles bigger as the muscles become warmer. Rotating the wrist as far as possible is a good way to increase the range of motion in the area.

2) Shoulder and Neck Stretches

People who do a lot of repetitive exercises as part of their work or hobby tend to develop a lot of tension in the shoulder and neck area. The same can also be said for people who spend a lot of time using a computer for activities such as gaming or people who spend a lot of time staring down at their screens sending text messages.

While a healthy person can get away with this for a while, it won't be long before they begin to develop pain in their neck and shoulders unless they make an effort to address this potential issue before it starts.

The best way to do this is to take regular breaks or change the action as often as possible to avoid staring down at the screen for too long. If tension has already accumulated in the neck and shoulder area then beginning these stretches and going for a regular massage session is a good way to avoid the problem getting any worse.

It is important to stretch out the neck area as any tightness in the neck can cause headaches and reduce the mobility in the shoulder region.

a) Neck Stretch

This is a good exercise to warm up the neck; the stretch should be felt down the side of the neck. A lot of people will probably be surprised to find out just how much tension can be felt in this area. If this is the case, then don't force the stretch, and only hold it for as long as it is comfortable. If any sharp pain is felt during the stretch, ease out of it.

Directions:

Tilt the neck gently to the left. Hold the stretch for three to five seconds and then repeat on the other side.

b) Neck Stretch on a ball

This exercise is especially good for excessive tightness in the neck region. It is performed lying down and the ball provides some resistance to stretch out against. Because of this, the stretch is more effective, however, it can also feel more intense so this exercise should be stopped the moment any discomfort is felt.

Place a ball under the neck; a medium sized ball with medium resistance is ideal for this. Gently turn the neck all of the way to the left, hold for a few seconds, and then return to the centre.

To complete the stretch, turn the neck to the right and hold for as long as is comfortable. This exercise can be repeated for a maximum of ten times, but start with small, gentle repetitions until the worst of the tension has been eased out.

The exercise can be repeated three to five times on both sides and can be done throughout the day to reduce and prevent tension from building up.

3) Shoulder Stretches and Relaxation

Anyone who spends a lot of time carrying out repetitive activities will be familiar with the dull ache in the shoulder muscles that can result due to overuse and tension. If this is allowed to continue then the symptoms will become more severe and can lead to the development of conditions such as tendinopathy or Repetitive Strain Injury.

Eventually, the pain might start to feel like a burning pain, a sure sign that there is inflammation in the tendons. If a patient has Carpal Tunnel Syndrome due to repetitive activity then it is likely that they will also have tightness in the shoulder muscles, so stretching these muscles out is important to stop the tension spreading.

One way of relaxing the shoulders it to use a massage cushion. Although they are not a replacement for massage therapy, these cushions are ideal for reducing the stress in the shoulder region and are helpful for people who carry out a lot of repetitive actions. The massage cushions are set to work for approximately twenty minutes at a time and there is an option of using heat to further enhance the relaxation process.

A heated massager can also be used, however it is more difficult to target the shoulder area with a massager, so targeted stretches that are designed to alleviate shoulder tension are much more effective.

a) Shoulder Stretch

This exercise will help to relax the shoulders and the top of the back. It is especially useful for people who do a lot of computer work or sit in one position for long periods of time.

The stretch can be carried out throughout the day and it will help to release the tightness that starts to build in the neck muscles as well.

Shoulder pain can also be common place in Carpal Tunnel Syndrome as a weakness in the wrists will mean the others muscles will need to work harder, so stretching out the shoulders is an excellent way to reduce any tension that might have gathered in the upper back and shoulder area.

Directions:

Interlink the fingers and stretch them out. As you relax into the stretch, curl your neck forward slightly to enhance the stretch in the shoulder area. This stretch will also be felt in the back of the neck.

The stretch should be held for 15-30 seconds and repeated on both sides. Office workers can benefit from doing this stretch as often as possible, and it is beneficial for occupations such as hairdressing as well.

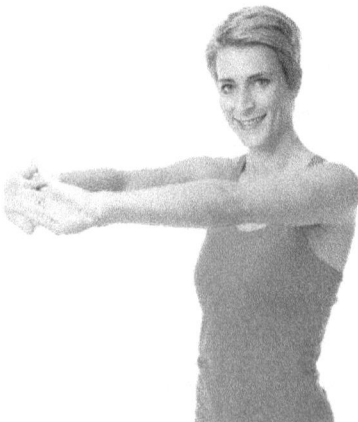

b) Shoulder Stretch 2

This exercise will help to stretch out the back of the shoulder.

Directions:

Extend your right arm in the air and then bend it down until it touches your right shoulder. Reach your left arm up and add some gentle pressure to the elbow to feel the stretch in the shoulder area.

The stretch should be repeated three times on each side and held for ten to thirty seconds each time.

Do this stretch whenever you feel tension gathering in the shoulders.

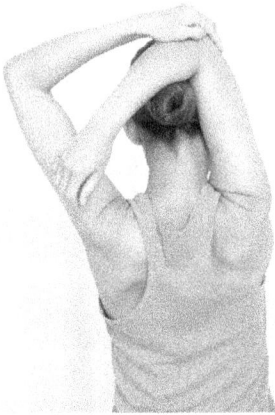

4) Strengthening Exercises

When it comes to building strength in the wrist area, it is best to work with a physiotherapist as they can better determine where the weakness lies. They can suggest exercises that will be suitable for the patient's needs and help to ensure that they don't overwork the muscles.

Avoiding overworking the muscles is essential, especially if this is what contributed to the development of Carpal Tunnel Syndrome in the first place. Moreover, a patient doesn't want to do any exercises that might make the pain worse, so take expert advice before beginning a strengthening programme.

a) Wrist, Arm and Shoulder Strengthening Exercises

Patients with Carpal Tunnel Syndrome might find using a resistant band easier to do muscle building exercises with. These bands are available in varying levels of resistance and give the muscles something to work against without putting too much stress on the muscles or joints. They also make sure that the load is even so that you don't work one side harder than the other, however, these exercises can also be carried out by using light weights, or with no weight at all to begin with.

b) Wrist Curls

This exercise focuses on building strength in the wrist and making everyday actions such as gripping easier.

Directions:

Begin by sitting up straight on a sturdy chair or on the bed with the feet flat on the ground. Hook the resistance band under the arches of the feet and then take hold of the ends of the band so you are holding one end in each hand; make sure that both sides of the band are of equal length.

Gently grip the resistance band as you gently curl your hand in towards you from the wrist, and then uncurl the wrist. Repeat the action as many times as it comfortable, and take care not to over work the wrist area; 3 to 5 times should be enough when starting out.

c) Bicep Curl

In the first chapter it was explained how it is important to build up strength in the other parts of the arm as these muscles will be required to take on an extra workload if there is a weakness lower down in the arm.

This simple exercise can help to build up the biceps. Begin in the same position as the previous exercise, with the resistance band hooked under the feet, the feet flat on the ground, and an equal length of the band in each hand. This time, curl the arm in from the bicep, wait a few seconds while you feel the contraction in the upper arm and then release. Repeat this move 3-5 times until you have built up strength and are able to do more without causing pain.

d) Triceps Toner

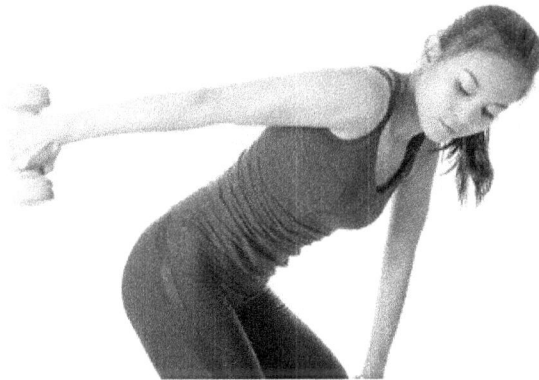

Muscles should always be worked in pairs, so once the biceps have been exercised, it is important to do the same with the triceps. This exercise can be performed with a resistance band, but it is easier to use light weights for this exercise.

Once these exercises have been completed, use some of the yoga exercises to stretch out the upper body muscles, or use some of the other stretches detailed in this chapter.

Directions:

Take a pair of handheld weights and stand up with one foot behind the other; the knees should be bent.

Lean forward and ensure that your spine is straight. Extend your arm behind you until you feel the contraction in the tricep muscle. Do the same amount of tricep exercises as you did of the bicep exercises.

e) Shoulder Raises

The following exercise helps to build up the shoulder area and maintain strength, however, if you have an on-going shoulder problem, suffer from tendonitis/tendinopathy, or if your shoulders are excessively tight, then don't attempt the exercise.

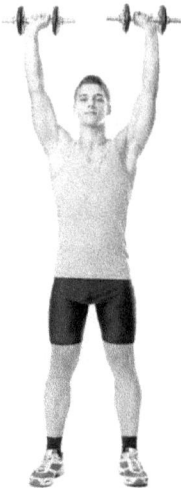

Directions:

Take a weight in each hand and slowly raise them above your head. Hold the move while you feel the contraction in the shoulders and then lower them.

If lifting the shoulders this high is too difficult then raise the arms to chest height instead.

Repeat the move three-five times until your strength has built up and remember to warm up the shoulder muscles and stretch them out afterwards.

5) Resistance Hand Exercisers

Resistance hand exercisers are also recommended for exercising the wrist area. They are suitable for patients with Carpal Tunnel Syndrome, arthritis and Repetitive Strain Injury; they come in a variety of strengths.

These exercisers can be used to gain and maintain strength in the wrist, build muscle and improve grip in the hands and improve circulation.

They are available from a wide range of manufacturers. Before purchasing, it is best to discuss this with a care team so they can help determine which product would be the most suitable for the patient.

There is one product that has been designed specifically for use by patients with Carpal Tunnel Syndrome and Repetitive Strain Injury. The Handmaster Plus by Doczac is a small exercise ball and is designed to strengthen the muscles in the hand, wrist and elbow. It can also be used by patients with tennis or golfer's elbow, to help rehabilitation after a sprain or fracture, and to strengthen the grip in patients with arthritis or who have suffered a stroke. In addition, it can be used during the post-surgery process or to build muscle in patients with a weak grip.

The ball comes with five finger loops that will attach to the ball; an instruction leaflet in the box illustrates the exercises that can be carried out by using the ball. However, using the ball on its own can also provide a good strengthening workout for the hand and wrist area and just doing this might be enough for patients who want to start building up weakened muscles in the hand and wrist area.

An alternative to the Handmaster plus is the Gripmaster. This comes in varying strengths; beginners should use the lightest one. It will develop strength in the wrist and forearm and will help to maintain dexterity. This device is particularly useful for patients who want to strengthen their fingers.

6) Stretches for Computer Users

Stretching helps to relax your muscles, so they are less likely to get injured. It also breaks up scar tissue that forms from RSIs, which promotes healing. Stretches feel good to most people, and re-energize them. Stretching should not hurt; never stretch to the point of pain. If these stretches are painful, you may already have an injury and should consult your doctor.

The Canadian Centre for Occupational Health and Safety recommends stretches like the following for computer users.

Shoulder Shrug

Raise the top of your shoulders toward your ears until you feel slight tension in your neck and shoulders. Hold for 3-5 seconds. Relax your shoulders and repeat 3 times.

Shoulder Roll 1

Sit down and make yourself as tall as possible. Slowly roll your shoulder to the back in a circular motion. Then roll your shoulders forward. Repeat 5 times each way.

Shoulder Roll 2

Stand up and put your hands at your side and relax your shoulders. Slowly roll your shoulders in a backwards and forewords direction and try to make the circle you make by rolling as large as possible. Repeat 5 times each way.

Shoulder Stretch

Sit down on a chair and put your hands behind your heads with your elbows pointing outwards. Push your elbows gently forward towards each other and try to stretch until the tips of your elbows touch. Hold for 5 seconds and repeat a few times.

Neck Stretcher 1

Drop your head slowly to the left, trying to touch your left shoulder with your left ear until you feel the stretch in the right side of your neck. Hold for 3 seconds Bring your head back to normal position. Drop your head slowly to the right, trying to touch your right shoulder with your right ear until you feel the stretch in the left side of your neck. Hold for 3 seconds. Bring your head back to normal position. Repeat 3 times each way.

Neck Stretcher 2

Drop your head slowly to the left, trying to touch your left shoulder with your left ear . Then, slowly drop your chin to your chest; turn your head all the way to the left, then all the way to the right. You should feel the stretch in your neck. Repeat 3 times and do the other side.

Neck Stretcher 3

Turn your head sideways as far as comfortable as you are looking to the left. Bend your neck over to look at the floor until you feel a stretch. Hold for 3 seconds. Return your head in original position and do the other side. Repeat 3 times.

Wrist Turns

Sit down and put your arms next to you. Turn your arms and wrist so that your palm faces outwards away from your body and then back inwards. Feel the stretch in your lower arm. Hold for 3 seconds. Repeat 3 times.

Upper Arm Stretcher

Sit down or stand up. Put your right arm forwards with the palm facing the floor. Now put your left hand underneath your right elbow and turn the palm of your right hand facing towards the left. With your left arm pull your right arm towards you so you can feel the stretch in your right upper arm. Hold for 3 seconds. Repeat 3 times with each arm.

Head turns

Drop your head down towards your chest as far as it feels comfortable. Turn your head left trying to look at your left upper arm and hold for 2 seconds. Turn your head right trying to look at your right upper arm and hold for 2 seconds. Repeat 5 times each side.

Back Curl and Leg Stretch

Hold onto your right shin with your right hand. Lift your right leg off the floor. Bend forward, curling your back, and bring your nose toward your knee. Repeat with the other leg.

Leg Stretcher

Sit on a chair and make yourself as tall as possible. Stretch one leg forwards and try to point your toes as far as possible towards you and hold for 5 seconds. You should feel the stretch throughout your whole leg. Repeat with the other leg. Do 3 times for each leg.

Forward lean

Sit on a chair and put your elbows and arms on your thighs and let your hands relax. Lean your head downwards. Sit like that and take 4 to 5 breaths and return in the sitting position.

Trunk Stretcher (the part of your body between your neck and your waist)

Sit on a chair and make yourself as tall as possible. Drop your arms by your side. Move your left hand towards the floor as far as you can but make sure that your trunk stays upright. Hold your arm for 5 seconds. Return to sitting position and repeat with right arm. Repeat with each arms 3 times.

Forearm Twist

Sit down on a chair and put your hands on your lap with the palms facing your legs. Relax your shoulders. Turn your hands so that your palm is now facing up. Gently push your thumbs outwards as far as comfortable and hold for 3 seconds. Turn your hand again to face your legs. Repeat with 5 times.

Stretch your arms and fingers

Sit on a chair and make yourself as tall as possible. Put both of your arms forwards with the palm of your hands facing you. Interlink your fingers. Roll your palms/arms so that they now face away from you. Stretch by reaching out as far as you can and hold for 5 seconds. Feel the stretch in lower arm and fingers. Repeat 3 times.

Stretch your arms and shoulders

Sit on a chair and make yourself as tall as possible. Put both of your arms forwards with the palm of your hands facing you. Interlink your fingers. Roll your palms/arms so that they now face away from you. Move your arms so they are now above your head. Stretch by reaching out as far as you can and hold for 5 seconds. Repeat 3 times.

7) Stretches for Texters

Yes, texting is a big problem and can lead to problems in the hand and the wrist.

Virgin Mobile and the British Chiropractic Association suggest stretches to reduce the risk of repetitive strain injury amongst people who are heavy texters. Use these exercises before and after texting and between texts if you are doing it for long periods of time. These stretches should not hurt. If they do, it's time to seek medical advice.

Thumb stretch

With the right palm facing down, hold the thumb of the right hand with the fingers of the left hand. Pull the thumb gently and hold for 10 seconds. Repeat three times, then reverse hands.

Arm stretch

Stretch your left arm in front of you, palm up. Place your right hand on top of the left with fingers and thumbs lined up. Point your fingers down and hold for 10 seconds. You should feel a gentle stretch on the inside of your left forearm/wrist. Repeat three times, then reverse hands.

Finger stretch

Hold hand out, palm down. Spread fingers and thumbs as far as you can. Hold 2-3 seconds. Then make a fist and hold 2-3 seconds. Repeat 3 times.

Arm and finger stretcher

Sit in a chair and make yourself as tall as possible. Lean back as far as you can so you are looking towards the ceiling. Spread your arms (like you did as a kid when you were flying an aeroplane) and rotate your arms left and right. Spread your fingers and thumbs out as much as possible. Repeat 2 times.

Chest stretch

Stand straight with your hands on your hips. Bring your elbows back, keeping your shoulders down. Get your elbows as close together as you can comfortably. Hold for 10 seconds and repeat three times. You should feel a stretch across your chest and/or shoulders.

Neck stretch

Pull the chin in slowly, trying to make a double chin. Hold for 2-3 seconds and repeat three times.

Shoulder stretch

Shrug your shoulders up toward your ears. Hold for 2-3 seconds, then relax. Repeat 3 times.

8) Yoga Exercises

Yoga exercises can be an extremely effective means of reducing pain in the shoulders, wrists, hand and fingers. However, some yoga instructors warn against practicing some of the yoga moves if the patient has wrist pain.

Yoga is also a good way of preventing problems such as RSI and Carpal Tunnel Syndrome as it helps to stretch out the upper body muscles and stops tension building in the first place.

Studies have also shown that that yoga can help reduce the pain caused by Carpal Tunnel Syndrome. Yoga can also help to improve grip and it is best practiced alongside a relaxation programme.

However, it is important to keep any undue pressure off of the wrist area when practicing yoga, so if any discomfort is felt then come out of the pose.

For all poses, make sure that you are dressed comfortably. There is no need for any special clothing, just wear something that you will be comfortable in such as loose trousers and a T-shirt. The postures should be practised without footwear, however, if you are diabetic, or if you suffer from poor circulation or numbness in your feet, then it is a good idea to wear yoga socks or yoga shoes to protect the feet.

a) Spinal Twist

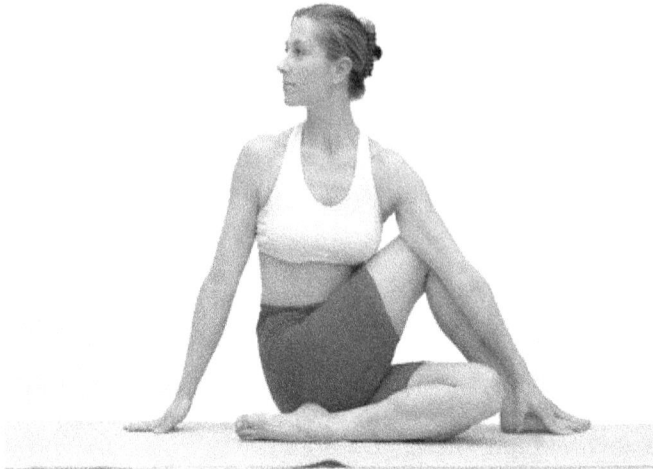

The spinal twist is a good exercise for releasing stress and pain in the lower back area and it is believed to be therapeutic for people suffering from Carpal Tunnel Syndrome.

When completing a spinal twist, make sure you keep the movements small and smooth as completing any movement that your body isn't used to can lead to injuries if you are not careful.

Begin by extending both legs out straight in front of you. Bend the left knee towards the body and rest it on the floor, then cross the right leg over.

With an inhale, extend the right arm up and bring it behind you, take a breath and with another inhale extend your left arm up and stretch it down so it rests against your front leg.

Gently turn your head to look over the shoulder and take five full breaths in and out. Then return to face the front. Repeat the move on the other side.

Precautions:

Patients with blood pressure problems, migraines or headaches should not attempt this move.

Alternatives:

The spinal twist can be completed by keeping one leg out straight and the other knee bent and the foot flat on the floor. Hook the opposite hand around the bent knee and then turn to look over your shoulder.

b) Spinal Twist on a Chair

For a much gentler version of this move, the spinal twist can be completed in a chair. The stretch will not feel as powerful, however, but it is a good place to start for beginners who want to start to build flexibility in their spine.

Directions:

Sit up straight in a chair and with both feet flat on the ground and the spine erect. Place one hand on the side of the chair and on an in breath turn to look over your shoulder. Make sure that the turn is gentle and take care not to make any sudden, sharp movements.

Repeat on the other side.

Once you have practiced the basic twist poses, there are several other spinal twists that can be mastered. These are all excellent at giving the spine a stretch and releasing tightness in the spinal column.

However, many of these poses are not for beginners and should not be practiced without expert tuition.

c) Forward Bend

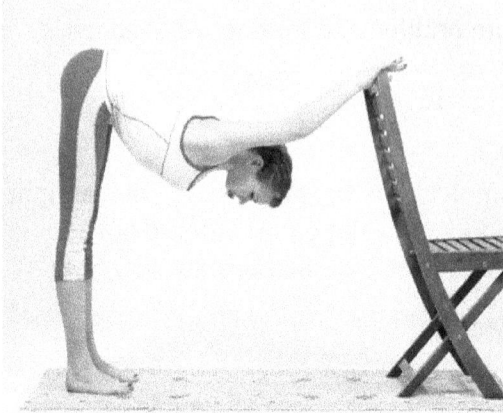

This is an easy alternative for those just starting out and who want a gentler stretch than the full forward bend. Choose a sturdy chair for performing this posture; you can also reach out to the seat of a chair if this feels more comfortable.

Begin by taking a few steps away from a chair; you just need to take enough steps away so that you can reach out and touch the chair without forcing.

With an inhale, extend your arms upwards and then reach them out to rest your hands on the top of the chair. Hold the pose for five breaths and come up with and inhale.

Precautions:

The forward bend helps to calm the body and the mind. However, it should not be practiced by patients who are suffering from problems with their blood pressure, headaches or migraines.

d) Downward Dog Pose

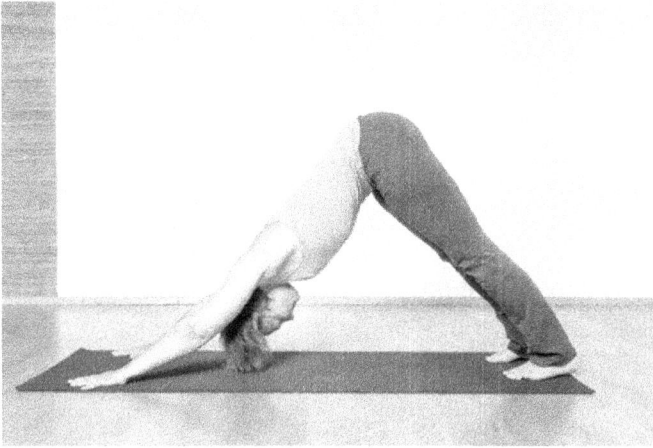

The Downward Dog Pose can be used on its own or as part of the Sun Salutation set of postures. The Downward Dog posture will stretch the Achilles and calves, your shoulders, wrists and your chest, and will also help to calm your mind.

It is an ideal posture for helping to prevent tendonitis and if practiced regularly, it can help prevent tightness and tension from building up in the wrist area. However, some yoga experts advise against practising this move if you already have wrist problems, so seek advice before practising this posture.

You can get into this posture by kneeling, then reaching your hands forward, breathe out and gradually lift your knees. Press your hands firmly into the ground and continue to straighten your hands and knees until you reach the inverted V position. Hold the position for five breaths and then come out of the pose by gently lowering your knees back down to the floor.

Precautions:

This posture should not be attempted by patients recovering from surgery for the wrist area. In addition, patients should be careful not to put too much weight on the wrists when they move into this posture.

For an easier alternative, and a gentler stretch, patients can reach out to a sturdy chair rather than lowering their upper body all the way down to the floor.

Care should be taken not to lock the knees or the elbows while in this posture. Avoid this move if you have wrist, shoulder, arm, back or hip problems.

If you suffer from high blood pressure or are prone to headaches or migraines then you should take medical advice before practising downward dog or any of the inverted postures.

Before attempting any of the yoga stretches or exercises featured in this chapter, speak to a member of your care team first so they can help you decide if yoga is a suitable method to help manage your Carpal Tunnel Syndrome.

e) Child Pose

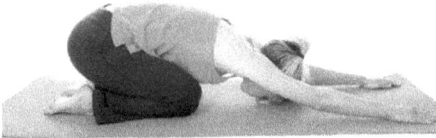

This pose is useful for stretching out the upper back and shoulder area. It is especially relaxing last thing at night as it will help to calm the mind and relax the muscles. It will also provide a stretch for the lower back area and is an ideal pose for people who have spent a long time sitting in front of computer.

f) Warrior Pose

The Warrior Pose is extremely effective for stretching out the upper body muscles, especially the shoulders and upper back. It will also provide a good stretch for the calves and legs and helps to strengthen the lower body muscles as well.

It is ideal for practicing at the end of a long day in front of the computer or after finishing any other repetitive action as it helps to relax and open up the upper body.

Precautions:

Patients with heart conditions or with high blood pressure should not do this pose. Patients with shoulder problems should take care when in this pose and not extend their arms above their head, and patients with neck pain should not look up while in this pose to avoid putting stress on the neck.

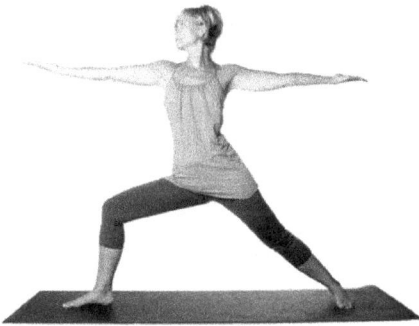

Directions:

Stand up straight and walk or jump your feet 2-3 feet apart. Turn your left foot to a right angle and your right foot pointing forwards.

Take an inhale and exhale as you move your right knee forward. Make sure that your right knee does not come over your toes or it will cause too much stress in the knee joint.

Hold the position for three to five seconds and then slowly come out of the pose.

g) Warrior Alternative

The hands can also be raised above the head while in the Warrior pose, but do not attempt this if you have shoulder or neck problems.

h) Eagle Pose

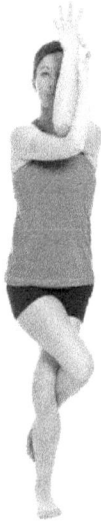

Eagle pose is a good pose for helping to release tension in the shoulders and upper back area. It will also provide a gentle stretch for the wrists if performed correctly, but take advice from your medical care team before doing this move if you are experiencing wrist pain.

The pose also helps to build strength in the lower body and improves balance; it will also help to improve focus and concentration. Eagle Pose can also performed sitting down, and just doing the upper body part of the pose.

Precautions:

Patients with hip or knee problems should be careful when practicing this move.

Directions:

Stand up straight and wrap your left leg around your right leg and sink your weight into the right side by bending slightly at the knee. Make sure you have your balance and focus on your breath. Make sure that you focus on a spot ahead of you to keep your balance and then wrap your left arm around your right wrist as shown in the picture on page 52.

Sufferer's story: *"I am 19. After texting my boyfriend 10 times, my thumb starts hurting. When I sit on my bed using my laptop, my neck is painful. I am so glad my friend wrote this book as she made me realise I have to look after my health better. I now call my boyfriend instead of texting him."* Source: my friend Georgina.

Chapter 9) Prevention

People can go a long way towards preventing the onset of Carpal Tunnel Syndrome. By following some basic tips you can learn some valuable advice on how to avoid Carpal Tunnel Syndrome. In addition, the following tips can help prevent the symptoms from getting worse.

However, the results will depend on how bad the symptoms of Carpal Tunnel Syndrome are and if the patient has any other underlying health condition that might be contributing to the CTS.

This chapter will highlight some of the main measures that a person can take to help themselves.

1) Splints

Splints are especially useful for people who do a lot of repetitive actions during the course of their work; typists and shop workers may find them particularly beneficial.

It is often recommended that the splints are worn at night to prevent the muscles from tightening up during sleep. However, they can also be worn during day-to-day repetitive activities.

There are a few things to consider before getting splints. First of all, a splint that isn't too rigid is best. Although it is important to wear a carpal tunnel splint that gives the wrist area some support, if the splint holds the hand so that it is rigid this can cause pain to develop in the shoulders.

Moreover, if splints are worn for too long, they can make the hands stiff so it is a matter of experimenting and finding a splint that is comfortable, that allows the hand to be functional without any tightening up of the wrist or hand, and that provides enough support.

When wearing the splint during the day, it is best to take it off regularly and give the hand muscles a stretch.

Splints are readily available and most popular sports' brands have their own version of them so it is a matter of doing some research and finding the one that works for the individual concerned.

If a patient is under the care of a GP or consultant for their Carpal Tunnel Syndrome then they should be able to get a brace from the NHS. However, these all tend to be made in the same way and might not be suitable for everyone.

Some patients might find it more beneficial to speak to a physiotherapist who can help suggest a brace that will be best suited to them.

2) Kinesiology Tape

During major sporting events, athletes can often be seen wearing coloured tape on their knees, ankles, wrists etc. This is kinesiology tape and it is designed to protect the joints as well as giving extra support to the muscles and tendons.

For some people, using this tape might be preferable to wearing a splint as it isn't so bulky, but also provides adequate support to the wrist area.

The tape can be removed and reapplied if necessary and will provide some light support to the wrist area. It can also be applied to the shoulder and elbow if these areas also get sore when carrying out repetitive actions.

When applying the tape, make sure that it doesn't meet completely and leave a small gap on the palm side of the hand. As with splints, using the tape can cause some stiffness in the wrist, especially if it is worn for long periods of time, so make sure to keep the wrist mobile and keep stretching at every opportunity to maintain flexibility in the wrist area.

3) Regular Breaks

When working on lengthy projects it can be tempting to keep on working until they are complete and it is easy to lose track time when doing repetitive actions.

The same can be said of many hand held devices. The constant sending of text messages, playing video games or consistently clicking on buttons on e-readers can all cause the repetitive stress that can, over time, lead to wrist, elbow and shoulder pain.

There is only one real answer to this problem and that is to take regular breaks. Take advantage of every opportunity that there is to stretch so that tension doesn't begin to build up in the wrist area and remember that the same actions that have caused your wrist pain can also go on to cause pain in the neck, shoulders, elbow and forearm.

If you are working from a computer and need to wait for downloads to complete, then this provides a good opportunity to stretch out. Alternatively, one of the therapy balls mentioned in the exercise chapter can be a useful tool for exercising the hands and changing the activity.

If it is feasible, place things that you are going to need somewhere else so you'll have to get up to get them, which will get you away from the computer. For instance, if you are working from home, keep any papers or notes that you are going to need in the room next to the office so you have to get up to go and get them. Not only does this give you the opportunity to stretch, but it is also healthier for you.

Sitting in front of a computer all day isn't good for anyone and the regular breaks will help prevent blood from pooling in the lower extremities and regularly stepping away from your computer will help give your eyes a rest and help prevent the tension headaches that can result as a part of eye strain.

4) A Balanced Lifestyle

While this might not be an obvious cause, studies have suggested that those who eat a poor diet, smoke or drink excessive alcohol might also be more prone to Carpal Tunnel Syndrome.

It is known that excessive drinking can cause peripheral neuropathy and poor nutrition can lead to dietary deficiencies that leave people more vulnerable to developing some types of neuropathy.

In addition, excess weight can also make a person more prone to Carpal Tunnel Syndrome.

If you are working in a stressful job, make sure that you get plenty of B vitamins, as stress can deplete levels of these vitamins; make sure your diet is nutrient-rich, including plenty of fruits, vegetables, salads, oily fish, nuts, seeds, and oils.

Make sure that you get plenty of exercise too, and if work doesn't permit this, then find ways of fitting it in to your daily schedule. For instance, park the car a little further away from the office or get out of the lift a floor early and climb a flight of stairs to get to your office. These are all practical things that anyone can do to include more activity into their daily routine.

5) Software

There is plenty of free software that has been designed to help boost productivity. However, this software can also be used to help prevent Carpal Tunnel Syndrome as it ensures that the user will get regular breaks.

One piece of software is called Install Boss. It is better suited for those who work from home and need to do a lot of typing as part of their job. Install Boss allows users to choose the amount of time they want to work for and a time for taking a break. For instance, you could choose to set the clock for 30 minutes of work and then have a two minute break – more if required – where you can do your stretches or other exercises.

A pop up window on this app will tell the user when they can take a break and when they can start working again.

Strict Workflow is another useful piece of software that works in much the same way. With Strict Workflow, the user can type for twenty five minutes before an alarm will sound; you'll then get a five-minute break before starting again.

6) Reducing Stress

Everyone will have different schedules so they will have different kinds of pressures and different tasks to fit into the working week, so it is essential that people take some time to look at their typical working and leisure activities across the week and see how they can reduce stress.

For instance, if you are always working close to a deadline, this can mean having to undertake a lot of repetitive work such as typing all at once in order to get it completed on time, which will cause a lot of stress on the upper limbs. Try to arrange your working time so that you allow yourself plenty of opportunity to complete projects without having to work close to a deadline.

Other actions such as clicking a computer mouse can also cause a lot of wrist pain; it will contribute to tennis elbow – or mouse click elbow, as some specialists are calling it.

Try and organise your time so you don't have to do too much clicking or scrolling, as this can be damaging to the wrists as well. For instance, if you check your emails several times a day, try and reduce this so you are not clicking on messages to open them so often – anything to give your wrists and hands a bit of a break and use voice commands for searching and other functions on your computer.

Free apps are available for this and later models of windows usually come with some dictation software. Click on the search box that you'll find in all programs on your laptop/desktop and type in "voice recognition", if this if offered on your computer then you'll find directions on how to install it and set it up for use. Alternatively, try dictation software such as Dragon.

Chapter 10) Prevention Through Technology

Repetitive motions from using the keyboard and mouse and awkward postures are major contributors to CTS. You can use features of your computer as well as ergonomically designed equipment to reduce keystrokes and mouse use and eliminate awkward postures.

1) Computer Features

Slow down the mouse to reduce muscle tension in the hand. In Control Panel, double-click on Mouse. Select Pointer Options. Under Pointer Speed, move the slider to the left to Slow. Click OK.

Reduce the number of clicks needed. From the Tools menu select Folder Options. On the General tab find 'Click items as follows' and choose 'Single click to open an item.'

Use keyboard shortcuts to reduce keystrokes and mouse use. To see shortcut keys, go to View/Toolbars/Customise/Options and click on 'show shortcut tips.'

Use AutoCorrect to reduce keystrokes. AutoCorrect not only corrects mistakes, it can also insert phrases and paragraphs you use frequently. Go to Tools/AutoCorrect. Add mistakes you commonly make and the corrections. You can also add phrases and assign them a shortcut phrase. For example, if you have a standard closing paragraph you use for letters, you can add that in AutoCorrect and give it a name, like "closing." Then all you have to type is "closing" and AutoCorrect types the rest.

2) Software

Voice recognition software allows you to operate your computer using just your voice. With hands-free computing your voice turns speech into text, so you don't have to use a keyboard or mouse. Dragon Naturally Speaking (http://www.dragonvoicerecognition.com/) and Talking Desktop (www.talkingdesktop.com/) are popular voice recognition software programs. Some Internet providers offer text-to-speech technology for reading and responding to email.

Break reminder software reminds you take a break if you go too long without one. Examples include

www.breakremindersoftware.com . www.workpace.com

3) Hardware

Alternative keyboards use various designs to help users keep their wrists straight, reducing their risk for RSIs. Split keyboards aim to straighten the wrists. Tented keyboards reduce the rotation of the forearms. Adjustable negative slope keyboards keep the hands from bending too far.

Before buying an alternative keyboard, make sure it is compatible with your computer. Then, try the keyboard for a few weeks before you decide if it works for you; it takes a week or two to get used to the differences.

The Goldtouch keyboard is a split keyboard that allows the user to position each section individually for maximum comfort. The Ergostars Saturnus keyboard is compact and easy to carry. You can learn more about these and other ergonomic keyboards at Keytools (http://www.keytools.co.uk/keyboards/) and at ErgonomicKeyboards.org (http://www.ergonomickeyboards.org/).

FrogPad (www.frogpad.com) is a wireless, Bluetooth, one-handed external keyboard that can be used with laptops, PDAs, and mobile phones. External and wireless, you can set the handheld or laptop at the right heights and angles.

Alternative mice relieve the awkward hand positions of most computer mice. A mouse shaped like a joystick is used vertically, positioning the hand more comfortably. Mice of different sizes fit larger and smaller hands. An ergonomic mouse supports the wrist in a neutral position. New designs in trackballs make them easier to use for people without fine motor skills. Keytools (http://www.keytools.co.uk/mice/), gizmag (http://www.gizmag.com/), and The Human Solution (http://www.thehumansolution.com/mice.html) offer selections of ergonomic mice, including hands' free mice for carpal tunnel syndrome sufferers.

Headmouse Extreme is a wireless head-pointing device that translates movements of the head into movements of the mouse. Designed for people who cannot use their hands, it is available from Liberator (http://www.liberator.co.uk/headmouse-extreme.html) and Techcess (http://www.techcess.co.uk/5_1_headmouse.php) . A programmable foot-controlled mouse (also called slipper mouse) takes all the pressure off the hands; sold through Amazon.com (http://www.amazon.co.uk/Foot-Mouse-Slipper-Programmable-Pedal/dp/B0061DVAOK) and Price Selector (http://uk.price-selector.net/search/foot%20pedal%20mouse?campid=5336926831).

Smartphones. Some newer models open up to a colour monitor and QWERTY keyboard that makes it easier to type with just two or three fingers.

PDA Stylus. Bigger styluses for PDAs are easier to grip. Papermate makes a 3-way pen/pencil/PDA stylus with a padded grip.

Sit/Stand Workstations. Workstations that let workers easily change from a sitting position to a standing position are becoming increasingly popular in schools, offices, and call centres. Ergotron (www.ergotron.com), GeekDesk (www.geekdesk.com/), and Nielsen (www.nielsen-associates.co.uk/sit-stand/) are three of many designers and manufacturers of height adjustable and sit/stand desks.

Scanners. Using a scanner is a practical and efficient way to reduce the amount of typing you have to do. You will need a scanner that has built in OCR software (Optical Character

Recognition). All you do is scan a page and it recognises all the characters and brings up the page into MsWord.

Cell Phones, Video Games and Other Hand Held Devices

4) The Hazards

With 93.5 million text messages being sent every day in the UK, RSIs from texting could become an epidemic. In response to a question on Yahoo, one texter said she sent over 8,000 text messages in one month (that's over 250 a day)! London-based Virgin Mobile reports that 38 percent of its frequent users have sore thumbs and wrists from texting. That's not all: each year 3.8 million people experience an injury related to texting.

Video games are a billion dollar industry with the amazing graphics and music but obviously from a commercial point of view the video games manufacturers are not telling you that overuse can affect your future.

Playing video games usually means hours of immobility and this prevents proper blood flow to the extremities. The spine can be curved unnaturally and become very painful as most people play games with a curved back.

Cell phones, video game consoles, and other hand held devices haven't been around long enough to see the kinds of long term problems they might cause. However, short-term health effects are becoming common enough to have their own names. "Text messaging injury" or "TMI" is pain and swelling of tendons at the base of the thumb and the wrists. It's common amongst young adults as well as working people who are tied to their jobs via texting. "Cell phone elbow" refers to pain, tingling, and numbness in the arm and forearm from bending the arm for long periods of time.

Texting Thumb, Nintento Thumb or Nintendinitis are now terms used often in the medical industry.

Looking at a typical handheld device, it's easy to see how it could cause a repetitive strain injury. The small size requires a tight grip, as does the tiny stylus of most PDAs. As the screen is so small, users hunch over to see it, bending their necks, stooping their shoulders, and rounding their backs. Clenching a phone between the ear and the shoulder requires even more neck bending. In fact, neck pain is the most common complaint of frequent cell phone users. Thumbing messages repeats the same small motions over and over resulting in TSI.

A study conducted in Taiwan measured the changes the body goes through during texting. Eighty-three percent of the study participants reported hand and neck pain whilst they were texting; plus, they held their breath when they received text messages.

5) Safer Use of Mobile Phones

You can reduce the risk of getting a RSI from a hand held device by paying attention to these safe practices:

\-   Hold the device in one hand and use the fingers of the other hand to type. Don't hold it in one hand and use the thumb of that hand for keying.

\-   Store commonly used numbers in the cell phone's address book to reduce the amount of keying you have to do.

\-   Use a headset for phone calls, or hold the phone in your hand.

\-   Switch sides every 10 minutes if you must cradle the phone between your ear and shoulder.

\-   Limit your texting to no more than 1½ hours in 24 hours.

\-   Use handheld devices for short messages only.

\-   If your hands start to hurt, stop texting and massage your arm from wrist to elbow.

-        Change position frequently and stretch your arms, shrug your shoulders, and move your fingers around to relax your muscles.

-        Try out new hand held devices before you buy them to make sure you can use them comfortably.

-        Use the predictive text feature of the mobile phone to reduce keystrokes.

-        Keep your shoulders relaxed, down away from your ears. Bring the device into your field of sight rather than bending your body to see it. Hold the device below the level of your heart and keep your back straight.

-        When using a device for tasks other than phone calls, keep elbows next to your body, bent at about 135 degrees. Keep your head straight and over your shoulders. Look down on the device without bringing your head forward.

6) Safer Use of Video games

There is no need to totally give up the fun of video games but here are some important tips that will help to prevent injury:

-        Don't sit with a "hunched back". However uncomfortable it may feel at the beginning try and sit with a straight back.

-        Just like the athletes warm up their muscles, it is important that you warm up your hands before starting to game. If you are playing electronic tennis, warm up your arms and elbows. Basically warm up the body parts you will be using most whilst gaming.

-        Don't put your hands very tightly around the controller as this can over tighten the tendons. Instead, hold the controller as light as possible in your hands and push the buttons gently (however excited you are getting with the game).

-       Take regular breaks. I spoke to teenagers who literally spend 3 hours on a game without any breaks! That is a Definite No! Pause the game at least every 30 minutes and go for a short walk have a drink, stretch your legs, etc.. just move!

-       Do some stretches on a regular basis - every 10 to 15 minutes or so. Just stretch your arms and legs forwards, raise your arms over your head, move your shoulders up and down.

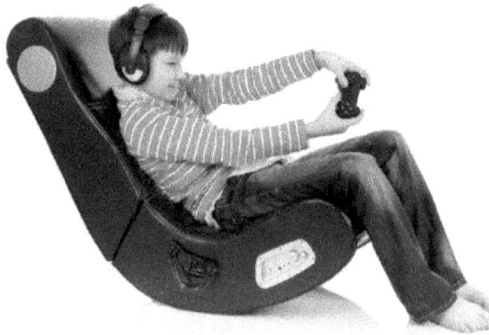

Chapter 11) A Word on Posture

The first step to creating a healthy work environment is good posture.

Good posture doesn't just relate to the positioning of the wrists when typing, but also to other areas of the upper body and in order to help manage or prevent the onset of Carpal Tunnel Syndrome, people must first learn the very basics of good posture.

As well as contributing to wrist pain, poor posture can cause problems with the forearm, shoulder, neck and back; it can also cause headaches.

People often get into bad posture habits and they don't always realise it until they notice the first symptoms of pain or irritation, but by being aware of how you are sitting and how you hold yourself as you move, it is possible to avoid some of the discomfort associated with poor posture.

Fixing the overall posture is essential to addressing the problems caused by Carpal Tunnel Syndrome.

1) The Problem with Sitting

Too much sitting is bad for your health. New research has found that excessive sitting may lead to obesity, type 2 diabetes, and heart disease. According to the American Cancer Society, women who sit for more than six hours a day are 37 percent more likely to die prematurely. Men are 18 percent more likely to die early if they sit too much. Medical professionals have long known that staying in one position for too long contributes to RSIs.

Furthermore, research concludes that vigorous exercise does not make up for long periods of sitting. That is, if you sit all day and then work out at the gym, you are still vulnerable to all the negative consequences of your sedentary day. Experts recommend frequent short breaks during the day to offset the sitting—active breaks where you move around. You don't have to stop working, just stop sitting.

Human bodies are built to move; when they don't, they suffer. Sitting causes the central nervous system to slow down, which leads to fatigue and sluggishness. Sitting weakens muscles and stiffens joints and as a result, posture gets distorted and the back and joints hurt.

When you sit at a desk typing, some of your muscles work too much and some work too little. This can result in painful muscles when you get off your chair or when you wake up in the morning. In just a short time of sitting, the body's electrical activity and blood circulation drop significantly. You can lose the ability to move. The body's effective use of insulin quickly goes down by 40 percent. The body burns calories at one-third its normal rate; just standing up triples the body's energy use. It doesn't take long for sitting to take its toll on the body.

James Levine, MD, PhD is an endocrinologist at the Mayo Clinic. He is responsible for some of the groundbreaking work on the effects of sitting, and concluded: "Excessive sitting is a lethal activity." Dr. Levine recommends standing desks because they let users make more small movements during the day than is possible when seated. You can buy a standing desk, but it's not hard to make one out of shelves or other furniture.

Dr. Levine designed (and uses) a treadmill desk, where the computer user walks at a very slow speed whilst working on a desk that surrounds the treadmill. Steelcase (http://www.steelcase.com) sells treadmill desks; Treadmill Desk (www.treadmill-desk.com/) has instructions for building your own.

Dr. Levine recommends lots of short, slow speed walks during the day. Here are simple ideas for incorporating walks into the workday:

- Stand up to talk on phone.

- Hold walking meetings. Walking meetings work best with two or three people and when there's no need to take notes.

- Talk to people in person. Walk over to co-workers to deliver messages.

- Make a walking track in the office. Outline a path with tape affixed to the floor.

- Take the stairs.

- Park away from the office; don't take the closest spot.

- Take a midday walk, saving half of your break time for eating lunch and half for walking.

- Use a standing desk or sit/stand desk.

2) Shoulders

Shoulder pain is extremely common in workers. As well as the repetitive actions that are carried out every day, there can be a number of factors that contribute to shoulder pain.

First of all, have a look at yourself in the mirror. Are your shoulders slumped or are they up close around your ears? Is one shoulder up higher than the other? If so then you are carrying tightness in the shoulders, which will often show as pain in the shoulders, neck and head.

If this is a problem area for you then try to consciously address it. Whenever you notice that you are holding tension in the shoulder region, make a conscious effort to relax it. One good way to alleviate this is to try some gentle stretches and another method is to try this simple exercise:

Sit down on a sturdy chair and bend over from the waist. Gently swing your shoulder from left to right without forcing the move or causing pain. The range of motion is likely to be limited at first; however, as you continue to do this exercise, it will get easier as the muscles will loosen. Tight muscles will cause pain, so this is an effective way to loosen up the tension and ease any aches.

3) Neck

Most people will have experienced pain in their neck after a long day sat at the desk. This is often because you'll be looking down at a computer screen or staring at paperwork, and this type of strain on the neck will also cause tension inbetween the shoulder blades. In addition, limited mobility in the neck area can also lead to symptoms of tingling and numbness in the fingers.

The first step to avoid this is to adjust the monitor height; you can read more about this in the chapter about ergonomics. The next step is to stretch regularly. There are some neck exercises in this book and these should be practiced throughout the day.

If you are experiencing head pain or a limited range of motion in the shoulder area, then it is likely that you have a neck spasm. If this is the case, then you'll need to speak to a physio as they can use a variety of massage techniques in order to reduce the spasm in this area.

4) Forearms

Proper positioning of the forearms is also important to prevent Carpal Tunnel Syndrome. The forearms should be kept in a neutral or flat position when typing, and not left elevated as they often are when completing computer work.

Typing with the forearms in an elevated position causes too much stress on the arms and the wrists. Forearm supports are available and they can help to support the lower arm area and make it easier to type for longer.

116

5) Finger Position

Finger position also needs to be addressed. Many people get into the habit of typing a certain way and they often won't notice the position their hands are held in, or realise the kind of stress that this can put on the wrist area.

Some people type with their hands pointing down at the keyboard with just the tips of the fingers coming in touch with the keys. This positioning of the hands is quite common in patients who have weak muscles in the wrist area and aren't able to extend their fingers/hands into a neutral position when they are typing.

Positioning the hands like this will cause excessive strain on the hands, fingers, wrists and shoulders, so if you notice pain throughout the arms and upper body area then check the position of the hands when you type.

Remember to occasionally watch how you type; if you notice that your fingers and hands are held in a pointed position when typing and you don't have the ability to pull them into a neutral position when typing then you could benefit from wearing splints or taping the wrist area to provide some support so that the hands can be held in a more neutral position, but this is something that should be discussed with your GP or consultant first.

Strengthening the wrist area can also help to ensure that the hands and fingers are held in a more neutral position when typing. If this is a problem for you, then speak to a physio who can advise you on the best kind of exercises for strengthening your hands.

The fingers can also have a tendency to tighten when doing a lot of typing and sometimes the tendons can shorten, giving the hands a "clawed" look. To try and avoid the fingers tightening up, stretch the hands and fingers as often as possible and use some hand therapy putty or a grip ball throughout the day.

6) Wrists

Many people put far too much pressure on their wrists when they type so make sure that there is plenty of space at your workstation so that the wrists can rest in a neutral or flat position on the desk when typing.

As detailed in the next chapter, wrist rests are available to help the wrists rest comfortably on the desk.

Sufferer's story: *"It pains me to write this – literally. My neck is crooked, one of my wrists feels like it has been trapped in a car door and there's a rapidly calcifying knot of nastiness lurking around my right shoulder blade... This is the price one pays for hammering a keyboard like Jerry Lee Lewis all day, every day for 15 years... Having blown all my wages on remedies, it seems the only real way to alleviate the ailment is to type less, which isn't easy when your entire working existence takes places electronically, you have book deadlines to meet and writing is all you can do. Source: Ben Myers in the Guardian 17 September 2010.*

What's the first thing that comes into your mind when you think about posture? For a lot of people the first thing they think of is standing ramrod straight without moving—like the guards at Buckingham Palace. Or maybe it's remembering grammar school and being scolded for squirming around in your seat and not sitting straight and still. With images like these it's no wonder many of us don't know what good posture really is—and don't really want to think about it either.

Good posture is about movement, not about being still. Pascarelli and Quilter define good posture as follows: "...good posture really means balanced use of muscles, ease of movement, and freedom from pain, not the tension that comes from holding yourself still. It is the ability to maintain proper alignment of the bones and length of the muscles through movement." Source: Repetitive Strain Injury: A Computer User's Guide

Awkward (or poor or faulty) posture is a major risk factor for repetitive strain injuries. Poor posture stresses the muscles of the neck and shoulder, sending them into spasm. The aggravated muscles can pinch the nerves of the upper body, causing pain and other symptoms.

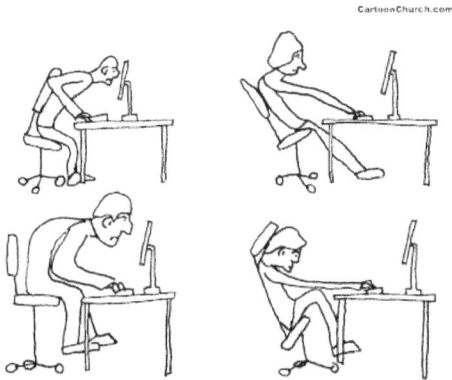

BAD POSTURE (EXAMPLES OF)

(Source: www.ergonomics-info.com)

Examples of Bad Posture

To understand the importance of the position of your hands when keying, try this: Holding your dominant hand with your thumb on top, grab a thick pen or similar object. Hold your hand in a neutral position (wrist, hand, and fingers in a straight line). Squeeze as tight as you can, then release. Now, grasp the item again and bend your wrist down, so your little finger moves closer to your wrist. (This position is called ulnar deviation.) Now squeeze. Can you feel how much more effort it takes to hold the pen tight? Now try it with your knuckles on top and your wrist bent back (extension), now with your wrist bent forward (flexion).

Most people find that it takes a whole lot more effort to hold onto the pen when the wrist is not in a neutral position, not aligned with the forearm and the hand. This is because the bending pinches the soft tissue and vessels, so it takes more effort. Think of it like a garden hose: when the hose is bent it takes more water pressure to get the same amount of water out. It's that extra effort, over time, that causes the small tears that add up to repetitive strain injuries.

Poor posture is hard to change, especially for people who are not particularly aware of their bodies or have been doing a job for a long time. A perfectly set up computer workstation can help users to hold their bodies properly, but it can't make them do it. Several of thetherapies discussed above, particularly the Alexander Technique, help people become more aware of their bodies and teach them how to put their bodies into alignment. It's not a bad idea to get postural assistance so you don't get a repetitive strain injury or CTS, rather than waiting until you do get one.

Chapter 12) Concerns for Children and Teenagers

Millions of children will be diagnosed, all over the world, with CTS, if they don't pay attention and look after their health.

1) A Growing Problem

Karen Jacobs, Chair of Ergonomics for Children and Educational Environment for the American Occupational Therapy Association and occupational therapist at Boston University, conducted a study of childhood musculoskeletal injuries from computer use. She describes the problem: "Computer-related discomfort in childhood and adolescence is of particular concern as the musculoskeletal system and posture are still developing…Young children worldwide are starting to complain now more than ever of musculoskeletal discomfort…" The point to remember is that because the heavy use of electronics starting at a young age is a new enough phenomenon , we don't know the long-term consequences. We do know that the consequences of early repetitive injuries can show up decades later, as the following story illustrates.

The problem of RSIs and CTS amongst youths is not limited to computer use. Game consoles, cell phones, and other gadgets put children at risk for injury. Kids get so involved in their games and projects that it's hard to tear them away from their electronics. An 11-year old boy in Scotland developed tendonitis from spending long periods of time on a Nintendo Gameboy, a condition half-jokingly called "Nintendonitis." Some students have so much pain and disability in their arms and hands that they cannot write their GCSE and A-level exam papers.

Surveys by the Pew Research Centre show that texting by teens is rising sharply. Between 2006 and 2009, the percent of U.S. teens who sent texts rose from 51 percent to 72 percent, an increase of nearly 50 percent in just three years. Half of teens send 50 or more texts *per day,* or 1,500 a month. Overall, girls send nearly three times more texts than boys. One-third of teens age 14-17 send over 100 a day (a practice called hyper-texting), for a whopping 3,000 texts per month. One U.S. teen sent over 9,000 text messages in one month!

The Chartered Society of Physiotherapy (CSP) in the UK warns that unless teens limit their texting they are likely to develop text message injury (TMI), which the organisation describes as pain and swelling of the tendons at the base of the wrist and thumb, which could create long-term injuries. Other research suggests that the more students text, the more pain they have in their shoulders and necks. (Makes you wonder about the necks, wrists, and shoulders of the competitors in the annual U.S. National Texting Championship sponsored by phone maker LG!)

Also worth noting but beyond the scope of this book is "toasted skin syndrome" or "laptop thigh" due to sitting with a hot laptop in the lap. The heat can cause mottling on young skin, and can lead to permanent darkening of the skin. Elevated scrotum temperatures, which can reduce sperm production and possibly lead to infertility, have been found in male laptop users.

2) Computers in Schools

According to Dr. Leon Straker of Australia's Curtin University of Technology School of Physiotherapy, nearly 90 percent of children enrolled in school in the U.S. use a computer at school and 60 percent of children in Australia who use laptops in school experience discomfort. He is concerned that back, neck, and shoulder pain amongst young computer users will develop into RSIs as the children mature.

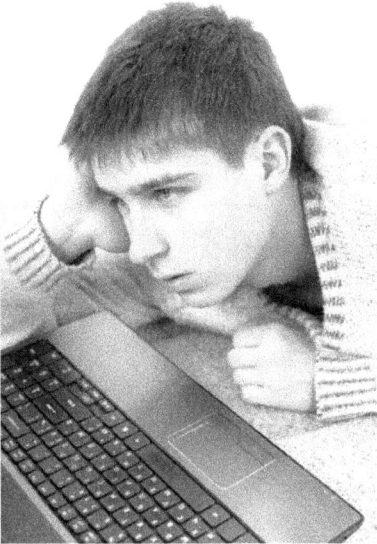

Typical wrong posture of teen laptop user

During its tour of schools in England the Body Action Campaign found the "vast majority using tables which cannot accommodate the range of pupil sizes, plastic bucket chairs and children with their legs dangling, shoulders hunched, without back support and head back gazing up at the screen." Researchers at Cornell University found that the computer equipment used by 40 percent of the U.S. school children they surveyed put the children at risk for postural problems in the future.

When providing computers for students, schools typically place the computers on existing desks, without considering proper workstation design or risks for RSIs. Schools that cannot afford new adjustable ergonomic furniture can adapt what they already have to make the users safe and comfortable. They can use stacks of books or reams of paper to elevate monitors and cardboard boxes or wooden blocks as footrests. Rolled up towels, jackets, or small pillows can provide lumbar support if they are anchored in place so they don't fall when the child moves around. Simple accessories such as these can be used to adjust the workstations to fit the wide-ranging sizes of elementary school children and promote sensible postures.

Where children use laptop computers at school they should be given external keyboards and mice. The external equipment will compensate for the lack of adjustability of laptops and make it easier for children to position themselves properly, without bending the wrists or holding the head forward.

Schools have the opportunity to teach children good computer work habits--habits that can help them avoid RSIs throughout their lives. It's hard to change habits later in life, so it's important to reach kids early. At a minimum, schoolchildren should be taught to:

-       Support their feet and lower back.

-       Lower their shoulders and relax their arms.

-       Keep their elbows level with the keyboard.

-       Keep their hands and wrists straight.

-       Bend their neck just slightly.

-       Keep their eyes level with the top of the screen.

CERGOS, Computer Ergonomics for Elementary School, has information and training activities for children and teachers at http://www.orosha.org/cergos/.

3) Computer Workstation Setup for Young People

Computer workstations for young people are not simply smaller versions of workstations for adults. Computer workstations should adapt to fit a range of sizes, because children change their shapes and sizes as they grow.

Desk Surface

The desk surface needs to be large enough for the keyboard and monitor to be side by side in front of the child.

The surface must be the right height so the child's wrists are straight with the elbows bent at about 90 degrees and the arms relaxed when keying. An adjustable height desk can keep up with a growing child and can be used by other people. Adjustable and sit/stand workstations make it easy for children to change positions.

Monitor

Place the monitor so the top is at or slightly below the child's eye level, directly in front of the child and about an arm's length away. Children should not have to bend their necks to look at their monitors. To avoid eyestrain, the image should be clear and stable and glare should be minimised by placing the monitor perpendicular to the window or using a glare screen.

Keyboard

Place the keyboard straight in front of the child, but away from the front edge of the desk to allow room for forearm support. Thin keyboards are better for children. For smaller children use keyboards without numeric keypads. The keyboard and mouse should be a little below elbow height.

Mouse

Place the mouse close to the keyboard; the child should not have to extend his or her arm to reach the mouse. A mouse bridge, which supports the mouse over the keypad, helps to keep the mouse closer. The mouse should fit the child's hand; use child-sized mice for smaller children.

Chair

If the chair and work surface are not height adjustable the chair needs to be changed to place the child at the proper height, that is, so hands and wrists are straight, the elbow is bent at 90 degrees, and the eyes are at or just below the top of the monitor.

The chair should allow the child's feet to rest flat on the floor. Otherwise, a footrest is needed. The chair should not have armrests. Lumbar support, if there is any, needs to fit the small of the child's back.

What do you think about the workstation below?

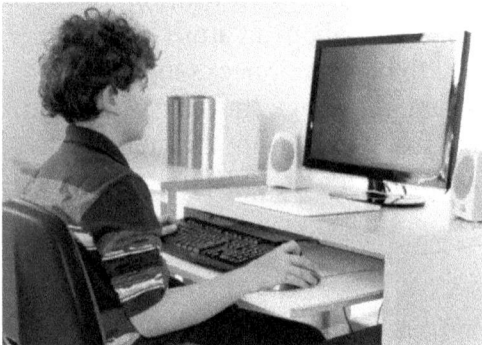

Good: Mouse close to keyboard, separate keyboard surface Bad: Edge of desk cutting into wrist, glare on screen, monitor too far back.

Improvements: Pad the edges of the keyboard surface. Raise the chair so that the elbows are closer to right angle (90 degrees). Raising the chair will also avoid resting arms on the desk, will improve hand position, and will move eyesight closer to the top of the screen. Add an anti- glare screen. Move monitor forward and closer to the child.

4) Laptops for Kids

Laptops should be used with a detached keyboard and mouse to allow children to position themselves reasonably.

Laptops should be carried in lightweight two-strap rucksacks instead of hanging off one shoulder. Rolled carrying cases are also good, but most young people don't like them.

Families may be able to modify adult-sized computer setups for young children. Another option is to buy kid-size monitors, keyboards, mice, and chairs. The following are among a growing number of companies that carry computer keyboards, mice, and furniture designed especially for children:

-       Ask Ergo Works, Inc. www.askergoworks.com/cart_ergo_kids.asp

-       Chester Creek Technologies. www.chestercreektech.com

-       Tiny Einsteins Computer Products. http://www.tinyeinsteins.com/kids_computer_products.html

-       QWERTY Keyboard, Computer Keyboards for Children. http://www.qwertykeyboard.org/computer-keyboards-for-children

-       Source 1 Ergonomics. http://source1ergonomics.com/

5) Stretches for Young Computer Users

The American Chiropractic Association recommends frequent breaks with stretches such as the following for young computer users.

Hand circles

Clench hands into fists and move them in circles inward and 10 circles outward—10 times inward and 10 times outward/

Hand squeeze

Place hands in the prayer position and squeeze them together for 10 seconds. Then point them downward and squeeze them together for 10 seconds.

Finger spread

Spread fingers apart and then close them one by one.

Wrap and twist

Stand and wrap arms around the body, then turn all the way to the left and then all the way to the right.

ErgoCoach is break and posture reminder software for children, with animated stretching exercises.
http://magnitudetechnology.com/productshome.asp

6) Safer Use of Electronic Gadgets

Electronic gadgets have their own hazards and risks for young people. One video game player described his painful experience: *"It's been hurting for like 4 months now. I am only 19 and I have the thumbs of a 60 year old...Got it from playing too much xbox..." And here's a similar posted on Twitter: "...got repetitive strain injury in my wrist from hardcore gaming Spyro. I regret nothing."*

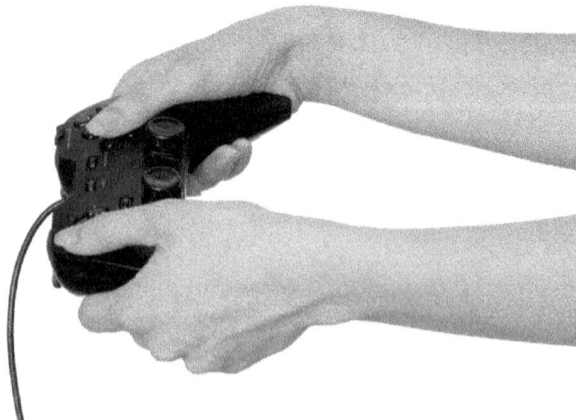

Teen operating game console. Note bent wrists and use of thumbs.

The 2010 winner of the U.S. national teen texting championship couldn't compete this year because of sore wrists. You shouldn't have to give up your gadgets to avoid injury. Here are ways to electronic devices and stay safe:

-       Limit the amount of time young people spend on electronic gadgets. CSP recommends limiting texting sessions to 10 minutes at a time.

        Spread the load by alternating fingers and hands when operating gadgets, including texting.

-       Avoid bending the neck back to look at game consoles.

-       Take frequent breaks to stretch and move around.

-       For children, use cell phones sized for small hands.

-       Buy cell phones for teens and young children that have parental controls that allow parents to limit calls and/or texting or that only allow a few pre-programmed voice calls. All phones for children and teens should have emergency call buttons and locator buttons.

Firefly (http://www.fireflymobile.com/) and Teddyfone (http://www.kiddyfone.com/) sell mobile phones designed for children.

Sprint Guardian is a bundled app service for Sprint. For customers on the family plan who use Android phones. Parents can lock their children's cell phones on demand or schedule locks for certain times of the day, such as during dinner, during school hours, and after bedtime. Guardian lets parents limit texting by their children and allows them to see the texts their kids send and receive. The service also has a locator tool. The "Drive First" feature automatically locks a teen's cell phone at speeds over 1.6 kilometres per hour (10 miles per hour). Sprint Guardian is a new service in the United States which is likely to prompt similar services elsewhere.

7) Teens at Work

About 80 percent of U.S. teens work some time during their school years. In the USA, teenage workers get injured at a higher rate than adult workers, even though child labour laws prohibit teens from doing some of the most dangerous jobs. In 2010, 20,000 teens got injured on the job, with 88 fatalities. Why is that? The high injury rate is probably due to teens' inexperience combined with their youth. They are new to the world of work and they may not recognize hazards on the job--like the hazards of working at a poorly designed computer station—nor do they know their rights as workers. Also, their youthful energy and desire to appear like adults may cause them to take unnecessary risks, to not ask questions and to not report problems. As a result of the current economic downturn there are fewer jobs for teens, so they may be reluctant to complain and risk losing their jobs.

Typically, neither school nor workplace prepares teens for working. Most schools do not teach workplace safety and health, and many employers don't provide the extra training and supervision teens need to do their jobs safely.

The National Institute for Occupational Safety and Health, or NIOSH, (http://www.cdc.gov/niosh/topics/youth/) has developed training materials and curricula for teaching youth about workplace safety and health. In keeping with teens' preferred method of learning, the NIOSH materials are visually engaging and specific to different industries. The materials address computer safety, as office work is a typical teen job.

Teaching teens about workplace safety and health before they start working is a good way to protect them from injury now and to prepare them for a safe working career.

Chapter 13) Ergonomics and Occupational Therapists

Proper ergonomics are essential for helping to prevent the onset of Carpal Tunnel Syndrome. A properly organised workspace is also important in order to reduce some of the stress that can be caused by repetitive actions.

If someone has already developed CTS then they are likely to need some help and support from an Occupational Therapist. In this next section, Debbie Amini explains how an occupational therapist can help in the treatment of CTS.

Conservative treatment (pre-surgical) provided by the occupational therapist includes wrist splinting, retrograde massage (in the case of swelling induced CTS), recommendation for isotoner glove wear (to reduce swelling if indicated), nerve gliding exercises (to prevent tissue adherent internal scaring due to tissue inflammation), carpal ligament stretching (to create more space within the tunnel, thus reducing pressure upon the nerve), and workplace or home activity modifications. If the condition continues to worsen or is not responsive to conservative measures, then surgery should be considered.

Occupational therapists can also see clients after surgery in order to provide and oversee a splinting program, address pain if present, increase motion, reduce scaring and improve strength and daily life function. If nerve sensitivity becomes problematic, therapists can also provide interventions to reduce hypersensitivity or provide a means of protecting the palm from pressure or touch (padded gloves).

Occupational therapists are, by training, experts in adapting the environment to enable function. This includes adapting the workplace environment (which may include home or school), to reduce the incidence of many types of work related disorders and injuries (of which CTS is one).

For a client who has early carpal tunnel syndrome, or one who is not seeking surgery, ergonomic modifications can be made to prevent or reduce symptoms. Since there are so many possible causes of CTS found in the workplace (positioning of the hand and wrist, force used for pinching, vibration, high repetition of job tasks), the therapist must first determine which of these risk factors is present and how it is impacting the client. Common adaptations include computer station modifications such as adjusting the height of the monitor, providing a wrist rest to place the wrists in a neutral position, adjustment of the chair and desk height to ensure a natural and relaxed position of the elbows, wrists and forearms.

In jobs that are highly repetitive, changes to tools or the manner in which a job is done may need to occur. Again, the therapist will need to see the job and ideally, the client completing the job in order to make appropriate recommendations. Sometimes a therapist may recommend that a job rotation program is started at the work site. In that way, each person only spends a few hours doing a repetitive task and then switches to one that uses different hand movements or positions.

Rest breaks are also encouraged every hour to enable changes in positions of the hands and wrists.

In jobs where poor positions are held for long periods of time, tools may be considered that will assist with holding, or height adjustments considered to place the arms and body in a position that will not create the need for awkward positioning. Again, rotating jobs and frequent rest breaks would also be encouraged. Adapted tools may also be used that decrease the need for awkward postures. For example, a drill that has a straight handle to enable a strong hold and direct downward force will keep the wrist straight versus a traditional electric drill with a pistal grip handle that must be used to drill straight down causing the wrist to deviate to the small finger and bend (thus cutting off blood to the nerve). Of course if drilling at a 90 degree angle, the pistol grip is the best choice. Multi-position tools are a good suggestion.

For clients that work with vibrating tools, products are available to dampen the vibration including covers that go onto the tool itself or padded gloves to dampen vibration at the hand.

When a client is required to pinch their thumb to their fingers using force or for long periods of time (taking notes, dental hygienists), adaptations are available including ergonomic tools to change the grip or support the fingers to ease the force required to hold the tool. For example, rubber tubing can be placed over a pen or pencil to increase the diameter, creating less focused force on the palm. Ergonomically designed pens will also lessen the force requirements needed to hold the pen for extended periods and can also improve wrist positioning.

Hand tools such as screwdrivers, hammers and pliers are now created with ergonomically designed handles and produced in multiple sizes that can be better matched to the size of the client. For example, smaller pliers will lessen the likelihood of several cumulative trauma problems including CTS for a female (or male) with small hands.

Higher technological solutions are also available for some jobs. For example, voice to text software will decrease the amount of typing that someone must do in a day. Laser mice will decrease the force needed to activate fields on the computer and roller ball mice will decrease wrist movement altogether.

Wrist splints can be suggested when they prevent movement or positioning that is problematic. It should be determined in advance if the client can use a splint at their job.

Client education is one of the most important things. If a client (with the help of the therapist) can determine the factors creating the CTS, they can likely think of ways to modify those factors.

Clients are the experts in their jobs and how they must be accomplished.

Returning to work following carpal tunnel surgery should be done at approximately 8-12 weeks depending upon the job setting. When needed, adjustments should be made to avoid pain. CTS should not recur, but nerve sensitivity may make a return difficult without attention to the work site. In addition, other conditions can occur.

Chapter 14) Organising the Workplace

Part 1) Office

The use of ergonomic equipment can greatly reduce the amount of stress and strain caused to the hand and the wrist while typing or carrying out other office duties.

Often it is not just the way that people type that puts a strain on their upper bodies; it's an accumulation of factors. Other issues that need to be addressed are poor posture and the height of the monitor etc.

This section will largely look at how to work more comfortably at a desk, however, for those people whose job involves repetitive activity such as factory work, then there should be guidelines available to help ensure that the employee doesn't go on to develop Carpal Tunnel Syndrome, and these guidelines should always be followed.

The following chapter will also address other areas of pain and discomfort that are common such as back, neck and shoulder problems. All of this needs to be addressed as they are often just another symptom of repetitive injury, and leaving these areas unaddressed will contribute to conditions such as Carpal Tunnel Syndrome. If a patient has been diagnosed with CTS due to overuse of their muscles/tendons, then it is likely that other areas of the body will have been put under similar strain too, so it's important not to just find a comfortable position for the wrists, but for the whole of the upper body.

For office workers, reorganising the work space can be helpful in reducing the risk of developing Carpal Tunnel Syndrome and if an office worker has already developed CTS, these tips might be helpful in preventing the symptoms from getting worse.

This next section will also include tips to help reduce other aches and pains that can be caused by office work.

Whether at home or at work, there are many ways to do repetitive tasks and avoid injury, including correct posture, ergonomic workstation design, safer work practices, stretching, and using technology.

1) Computer Workstation Setup

The term "ergonomics" has been thrown around a lot in the past 20 years. Ergonomics is about the relationship between people and the work that they do. Ergonomics focuses on fitting jobs to the people performing them, because when you try the reverse— fitting people to their jobs—you get injuries, illnesses, and errors. By designing workstations properly, ergonomics plays an important role in repetitive strain injury prevention. Ergonomics is also useful for accommodating people with RSIs so they can work without risking further injury.

A poorly arranged workstation makes it difficult to work in a comfortable position. By setting up your workstation correctly, you can make it easier to maintain a safe range of postures.

You don't have to buy new furniture if you can modify what you have to allow comfort and maintain a reasonable posture. The following specifications provide the parameters for a good ergonomic workstation.

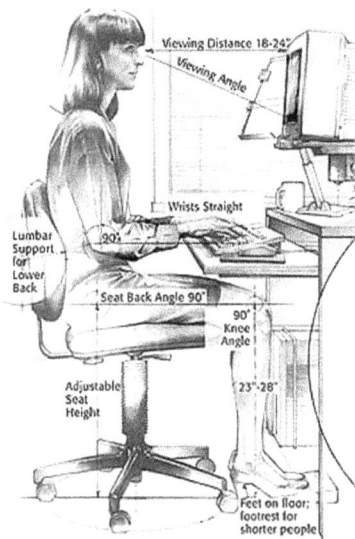

Ergonomic Workstation Setup

(Source: www.ergonomics-info.com)

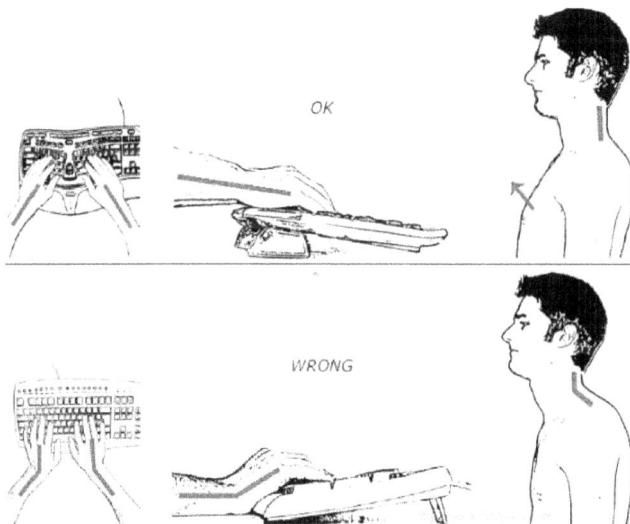

Source : www.rispain.com

2) Desk Surface

The desk surface needs to be large enough to place the monitor directly in front of you and at least 20 inches away.

An adjustable height desk will allow you to change positions and let other people use the computer comfortably. Sit/stand desks let users change from sitting to standing.

Leave plenty of room under the desk for your legs, feet, and thighs.

If the desk surface has a hard edge, pad the edges (for example, with pipe insulation) to avoid constricting your wrists.

3) Monitor

Place the monitor directly in front of you so your head, neck and body face directly forward when you look at the screen. If you work mostly from printed documents, place the monitor slightly to the side and keep the printed material in front of you, as close to the monitor as possible. Use a document holder to keep the printed material at the same level as the monitor.

Place the monitor 20-40 inches from the user. You should be able to read text easily with your head and body upright and your back supported by your chair.

Position the top of the screen at or just below eye level. Bifocal users may have to lower the monitor or raise the height of the chair to be able to view the monitor without bending the neck.

Position the monitor at right angles to windows to reduce glare. Glare is where sun light or a light shines on the monitor, making it more difficult to read the text on the monitor. Use an anti-glare screen if necessary.

Another good idea is to use two screens (see picture below) for example, one for your e-mails and the second for other work. This will keep your head and neck from staying in one position all day. All you need is a cable and software to install the second screen.

One University professor uses one screen for grading papers and another for everything else. In addition to relieving pressure on her head and neck, this system is more efficient, which means less time on the computer overall. Identical flat screens make the transition from one screen to the other easier.

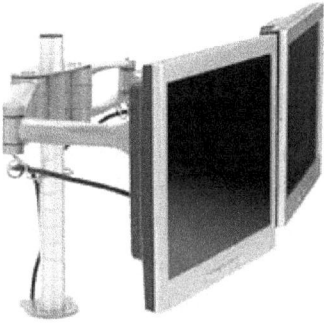

Monitor height is important for workers as they can develop neck pain if the monitor is not at the correct height.

Make sure that the computer screen is at eye level to avoid having to look down at it. Staring down at a computer monitor can cause excessive strain in the back of the neck.

If neck strain becomes too much of a problem it can cause spasms in the neck muscles. Not only can these spasms be very painful, they can also begin to limit the range of motion in the shoulder muscles.

Monitor risers are available and there are a range of gadgets available to lift a laptop so it is at eye level when you type.

Another key problem for today's computer users are netbooks and handheld devices. These are often used for leisure work, but staring down at the smaller screen will put too much pressure on the neck. The neck needs to support the head, which is extremely heavy and causes a lot of strain on the neck, hence the reason many people experience neck pain after staring down at their netbook all evening. Try using a netbook table to bring the netbook screen up to the eye level.

The need to be in constant contact is also a reason why many people are prone to repetitive strain injuries such as Carpal Tunnel Syndrome and RSI, as handheld gadgets and small screens put the same amount of strain on the wrists and hands, so look at ways to modify the use of these gadgets and take the time to stretch out the wrists and hands before pain develops.

Moreover, if Carpal Tunnel Syndrome is a problem for you, talk to your employer about how you can adapt your work load to avoid any unnecessary stress on your wrists, hands and shoulders.

4) Typing Position

Typing position is important to avoid strain in the wrists, fingers, forearm, elbows and shoulders.

As many people now use laptops to work from, this can contribute to the strain caused to the lower body. For instance, when typing on a laptop, the lower arms often don't have anything to rest on, leaving them without any support. This position is almost guaranteed to cause pain in the wrists, forearms and shoulders.

In order to prevent this, use a pillow or cushion to rest the forearms on when typing or use an ergonomic keyboard. These should be compatible with most laptops, and will make typing for long periods much more comfortable.

5) Ergonomic Chairs

A good chair for a computer workstation should promote good posture and allow for a range of positions. There's no single chair that's right for everyone, but there are common characteristics of a good ergonomic chair. An adjustable chair offers the most options for positioning for comfort. It's a good idea to try several chairs before selecting one.

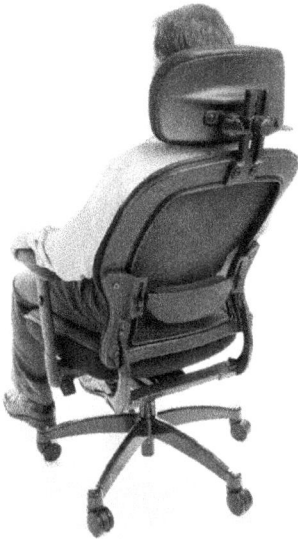

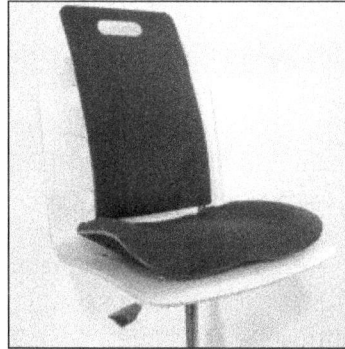

Adjustable office chair with lumbar support and 5-point base and next to it an ergonomic back support that can also help.

Here are the recommendations for a standard ergonomic office chair:

-        Seat height. Some "adjustable" chairs are so hard to adjust it's not worth the effort. An easily adjustable chair will have a pneumatic lever that changes the seat height from about 40 to 53 cm from the ground. Your feet should be flat on the floor when sitting in the chair. If you can't adjust the chair so your feet are flat on the floor, use a stable footrest. Many people use a footrest even if their feet reach the floor; it keeps blood circulating in the legs.

-        Seat pan. A seat pan (the part you sit on) between 43 and 50 cm wide is good for most users. Larger users may need chairs with larger seat pans. The front to back depth should allow the user to sit against the backrest and have about 7½ cm between the back of the knees and the front of the seat pan. The tilt of the seat pan should be easily adjustable. The seat pan should be padded and have a rounded (waterfall) edge.

-        Lumbar support. The lumbar support is in the outward curve of the backrest, which should fit into the small of the back.

-        Backrest. The backrest may be separate from the seat or attached to the seat. If it's separate, the height and angle should be adjustable and should lock in place.

-        Armrests. Armrests are optional (but not recommended for children). Your arms should not be on the armrests when typing. Armrests should be soft and adjusted to your shoulders so that they relax . Keep your elbow close to your body.

-        Base. A five-point base with casters makes the chair stable and easy to move.

Alternative types of office chairs may take some getting used to, but they can be worth the effort, especially for people with lower back pain.

-        Ergonomic stool. Ergonomic stools are designed to help computer users sit in a good posture. Stools support the low back and prevent sitting in a hunched position. The seat platform should allow motion in all four directions and should allow the user to sit at the height that is right for him or her.

-        Kneeling chair. Sitting in a modified kneeling position with no backrest slides the hips forward and aligns the back, neck, and shoulders. By distributing the weight between the pelvis and knees, this chair relieves the stress on the lower back. The kneeling chair makes it easy to maintain a safe and comfortable posture.

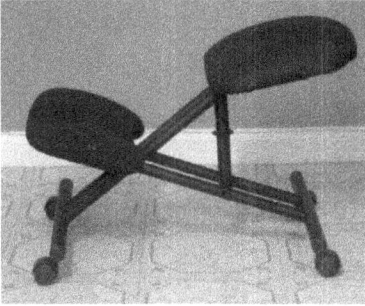

-

-         Kneeling Chair Source:
http://upload.wikimedia.org/wikipedia/commons/f/fb/Kneeling_c
hair.jpg

-         Exercise Ball Chair. This unique seat is a big round ball.
The slight bouncing of the ball keeps the legs moving, which
keeps circulation going and muscles active.

Ergonomic chairs come in a wide range of styles and are
reasonably priced. If you are only going to make one or two
adaptions to your workspace, then the ergonomic chair should be
one of them.

Before purchasing, you'll want to ensure that you are going to
purchase the right one for you, because if you purchase an
ergonomic chair that isn't suitable for your condition, then you
risk making any pain worse.

It is best to consult an occupational therapist who understands
your condition and how it affects you. They will be able to make
suggestions on which model would be most suitable for you. If
you are unable to get a referral to an occupational therapist, then
consult a physiotherapist who will be able to give you the best
advice on the model to buy.

Don't depend on other people's reviews when buying an
ergonomic chair, as what works for one person might not work for
another. However, a chair with a supportive back is a must if you

want to prevent back ache from leaning over the desk and arm rests will help to reduce stress in the lower arm area.

6) Foot Rests

Foot rests are ideal for taking the discomfort out of sitting at a desk for long periods of time. If you are sitting all day, this can put a lot of stress on the upper thigh area and can cause lower back pain.

A foot rest will help to keep your feet flat on the ground while providing support to the lower back and upper thigh area. Ideally, you'll want one that is adjustable so you can alter it until you find the most comfortable position.

7) Adjustable Desk

The height of the desk can also contribute to aches and pains. If the desk is too low then you'll likely to be hunched over it, which can cause pain and tension in the back and inbetween the shoulder blades.

If the desk is too high, you might find that you have to reach for the computer, which means your lower arms aren't supported and you are likely to feel pain in the hands, wrists and shoulders after typing for a long period of time.

The type of adjustable desk you need will depend on where your desk is positioned in the home or office and which tasks you use the desk for.

8) Back Cushion

Some people find ergonomic chairs a little hard going – especially if they have got into bad habits and they are used to slumping in front of the computer all day.

While adjusting to a new sitting position, you might find that you start to develop pain in the lower back, or you might feel some discomfort elsewhere in your body while you adjust to your new sitting position.

In order to make the transition from your usual work chair to an ergonomic chair, a lower back support can be very beneficial and help to reduce the initial discomfort.

9) Ergonomic Keyboards

There are many different models of ergonomic keyboards. There are some very basic models that cost less than £20 and much more advanced models that cost more than £200.

These are best purchased from specialist stores, as they have staff who can advise you on the most suitable model, as people's requirements will vary. However, there are models available for less than £10, and these could be worthwhile testing out to see if they are suited to your needs.

Most keyboards will require a USB connection to connect with your computer, so make sure that you have a spare USB slot that you can use.

If you can afford to buy a ergonomic keyboard, put the keyboard directly in front of you. Your shoulders should be relaxed and your elbows close to your body, about the same height as the keyboard. Your wrists should be in a neutral position (straight) and in line with your forearms.

Adjust your chair and work surface height as needed to achieve this position. If you cannot adjust them enough, use an adjustable keyboard tray.

10) Ergonomic Wrist Rests

The wrists need to be held in a neutral position when typing. If they are not, this can lead to compression in the nerves and thus lead to the development of the symptoms of Carpal Tunnel Syndrome.

An ergonomic wrist pad can go a long way to reducing discomfort in the wrist area. These rests attach to the wrist area and provide cushioning to stop the wrists from resting against hard surfaces such as desks. They can also protect the wrist area from resting directly against the hard edges of a keyboard.

Wrist rests that don't need to be worn are also available. These typically come with some gel cushioning and give your wrists a comfortable place to rest on, thus reducing discomfort from pressure points.

They are available as pads, long stick wrist rests, and in a variety of other models, so it is just a matter of finding the model suitable for you.

11) Ergonomic Mouse

Constantly clicking on a computer mouse can be another contributor to the development of wrist pain. A lot of people won't realise just how much the constant clicking of a mouse can cause stress in the wrist area; it can also lead to elbow and forearm pain.

However, an ergonomic mouse can serve to reduce a lot of this pain. They are available in a range of different models and price ranges and require a USB connection.

Finding an ergonomic mouse suitable for your use will depend largely on your hand size. People with small hands will want to choose the smaller devices as they will be easier to handle.

Again, it is advisable to speak to a specialist store, a physio or an occupational therapist before buying a mouse to ensure that the model is going to be the best mouse for managing Carpal Tunnel Syndrome.

If you can't afford an ergonomic mouse, keep the mouse (or other pointing device) close to the keyboard.

Position the mouse/pointer so your wrists can stay in a neutral (that is, straight) position. A wrist or palm rest can help maintain a neutral position.

If the desk or keyboard tray is not large enough for both the keyboard and the mouse, put a mouse tray next to the keyboard tray or a mouse platform above the numeric keypad.

Choose a mouse that fits your hand and that you can use without bending your wrist. Try different types of pointing devices, such as a touchpad, trackball, or fingertip joystick, to find one that is comfortable and suitable for you.

Do not grip the mouse/pointer tightly. Adjust the sensitivity and speed so you can control it with a light touch.

Use keyboard shortcuts to reduce the use of the mouse.

Alternate hands to give each hand a rest from mousing.

If you can afford it, buy an ergonomic mouse, just search for it on the web and you will find loads. Here's just one example:

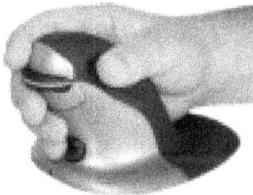

12) Ergonomic Tools

Working in construction or gardening can be another area that leaves people more vulnerable to Carpal Tunnel Syndrome. In order to help prevent this, or to make working more comfortable if you already have the symptoms of CTS, there are also many ergonomic construction tools and gardening tools available.

In addition, the use of wrist splits or braces will help to give some extra support to the area.

13) Sleeping Positions

A proper sleeping position is also imperative for helping to avoid upper body pain. If someone is spending eight hours a night not sleeping in a comfortable position, then this will add tension to the upper body area. The shoulders, neck, upper and lower back and wrists can all accumulate tension at night and can mean a person wakes up in pain, and then the discomfort and tension gets added to during other activities throughout the day.

By adjusting the sleeping position, it is possible to reduce a lot of this tension thus reduce some of the pain. For instance, if you already have pain in the arms, wrists or shoulders, try not to sleep on the affected side.

Make sure that you have a supportive mattress to rest against at night. Some people like the memory foam mattresses as they will conform to the person's natural sleeping position, however, others find them difficult to sleep on as they can feel hard when compared with other mattresses.

Memory foam pillows might also be worth considering if you have a neck or shoulder problem, however, while many people find benefits from using these, others find them too uncomfortable and they do take a bit of getting used to.

If you have been diagnosed with CTS, it is often advised to wear the splints at night. This will prevent the wrist area from tightening up overnight and will provide some support should you find that you sleep with too much weight on the wrist.

14) Avoid Eye Strain

Anyone who has spent a long time in front of the computer will know the feeling of eye strain. This can leave the computer user feeling overtired, with tired eyes and maybe headaches and neck pain.

Eye strain can also lead to problems with concentrating and make it difficult to read what has been written. This can in turn lead to people having to go back over their work to correct typos and re-writing sections of their work, which is all extra stress for the wrists, hands, and fingers.

To try and keep eye strain at a minimum, follow these simple tips:

Firstly, take a break from staring at the screen at least every twenty minutes. Take a moment to blink, rest your eyes, or look over to the distance – anything to give your eyes a rest and keep them from getting strained.

Use an eye wash or eye drops to keep the eyes fresh. This will also stop them from getting gritty or irritable, but take advice if you have diabetes or any eye condition before using drops or washes.

There are many natural eyewash products, which are made with ingredients such as eyebright; these are probably the best option for healthy eyes.

If you have dry eyes, which can sometimes cause blurred vision and add to eye strain, try some artificial tear drops. If you don't want to apply the tear drops directly to the eye, then apply them to the eyelids and underneath the eye area before massaging them in.

Adjusting the computer screen is also important to help avoid eyestrain. Try dimming the monitor, or add a screen over it. Screens are available to stick over the computer monitor and reduce the glare.

Gaming glasses are another effective way of taking the glare away from the screen. These are usually yellow tinted and can be quite expensive. Driving classes also come with yellow tinted lenses and these can be useful in reducing computer glare.

An optician can also prescribe tinted lenses. They might prescribe yellow tinted lenses or blue tinted ones, depending on your needs.

Pinhole glasses are another good way of resting the eyes – although you might want to reserve these for your leisure time or when you are on your own, as they don't look great, but they do reduce the headaches and help to improve the eyesight.

Lighting is also important when it comes to avoiding eye strain. Flickering lights will contribute to eyestrain. Products like Biobulbs are a good lighting option; they provide flicker-free lighting and are designed to appear like normal daylight, so they help to avoid eye strain.

For Break Reminder Software for your PC or laptop, visit:

www.breakremindersoftware.com

(only available for PC, not Apple)

www.workpace.com is more sophisticated break reminder software, available for Apple and PC.

15) Computer Workstation Checklist:

Checklists are easy-to-use assessment tools. The following checklist for computer workstations is adapted from the U.S. Occupational Safety and Health Administration (OSHA). Use it to find out if your workstation is set up properly. For any item you cannot check off, refer to the Computer Station Setup section for ideas on correcting the situation.

Posture

- Head, neck, and torso are upright—not bent down or back.

- Head, neck, and torso face forward—not twisted.

- Shoulders and upper arms are in line with the torso, about perpendicular to the floor and relaxed –not raised or stretched forward.

- Upper arms and elbows are close to the body—not extended forward.

- Forearms, wrists, and hands are straight and in line, with the forearm at about 90 degrees to the upper arm.

- Wrists and hands are straight—not bent up, down, or sideways.

- Thighs are parallel to the floor with lower legs perpendicular to the floor. Thighs may be raised slightly above knees.

- Feet rest flat on the floor or on a stable footrest.

Chair

- Backrest provides support for lower back (lumbar area)

- Seat pan is the right size for the user.

- Seat front does not press against the back of the knees and lower legs.

- Seat is cushioned, with a rounded front—no sharp edges.

- Armrests, if used, support both forearms and do not interfere with movement.

Keyboard and Mouse

- Surface is stable and large enough to hold a keyboard and mouse (or other input device).

- Input device is right next to the keyboard so it can be used without reaching.

- Input device is easy to use and fits the hand

- Wrists or hands do not rest on sharp edges.

Monitor

- Top of the screen is at or slightly below eye level, so it can be read without bending the head or neck.

- Monitor is at a distance so you don't have to lean your head, neck, or torso backward or forward to read the screen.

- Monitor is positioned directly in front of user—no twisting of the head or neck needed to see the monitor.

- Glare is not reflected on the screen.

- Screen is free of dirt and dust.

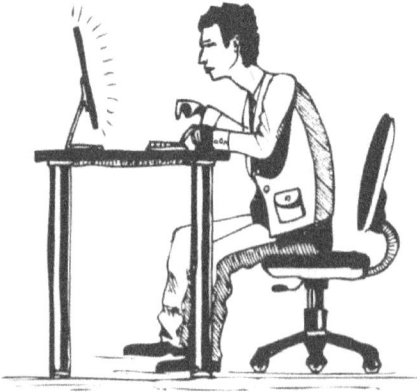

Head and neck bent forward because screen is too far away

Work Area

- Top of thighs have enough clearance under the work surface.

- Legs and feet have enough clearance under the work surface to allow user to get close enough to the keyboard and input device.

General

- Workstation and equipment can be adjusted so user can change positions and be safe and comfortable.

- Workstation has enough space to access needed supplies and documents without reaching.

- Computer tasks are organized to allow alternating with other tasks as well as adequate break.

Part 2) Other occupations/artists/crafts

Artists can also develop Carpal Tunnel Syndrome. However, there are tools available to help reduce the stress on the wrist and lower arm area. For instance, there are paintbrushes available with much wider handles to allow a more comfortable grip.

If crafts like knitting and crochet form a regular part of your working life or a hobby, then there are ergonomic needles and crochet hooks available that lessen the strain on the hands and wrists.

If using tools for a hobby or a job such as jewellery making, then there are many ergonomic tools available. These often come with spring-loaded handles and a soft grip to help reduce repeated stress on the hands.

Items like scissors, crafts knives and other essential craft tools are also available in ergonomic designs so people can continue their hobby or employment without adding too much extra stress to their hands.

1) Hairdressing

Hairdressing is another industry where repetitive strain injury can be a problem. Hairdressers often find themselves developing pain in their wrists, hands, forearms, etc. as a result of the repetitive stress that is part of their occupation. This can also be coupled with lower back pain from constant standing and neck pain from leaning over to wash people's hair.

Ergonomic hairdressing tolls are available, along with adjustable sinks to reduce neck pain.

As with other occupations that involve repetitive tasks, hairdressers should stretch regularly, break up repetitive actions by changing the way the tools are gripped or by changing the action.

2) Leisure Time

Many people don't associate their Carpal Tunnel Syndrome or the Repetitive Strain Injury with their leisure activities, but when the same action is completed repeatedly it has exactly the same impact on the body and can eventually lead to pain and tenderness.

One of the most common causes of RSI these days is playing computer games or texting. If you are constantly texting or spending hour upon hour in front of a computer game, don't be surprised if your wrists start to ache or you start to develop numbness or tingling in the fingers.

Take the same approach as you would in the work place and take regular breaks, do plenty of stretching and take time out to look away from the screen as often as you can.

RSI-sufferer's story: *I work at home on a laptop and have been having constant pain between the shoulder blades for some time, despite having an adjustable chair, and despite doing my best to sit up straight. Today I put my laptop on a cupboard - about waist height and added a couple of books to raise it a bit more. So far, it is a massive improvement.* (From Fishing Genet, commenting on a Guardian article at http://www.guardian.co.uk/society/us-news-blog/2012/jul/10/scientists-sitting-is-bad-for-you)

Chapter 15) Risk Assessment

1) Identifying Hazards and Risks

Risk assessment involves identifying hazards (things that can cause harm), the chances of being injured or made ill by the hazards, and the seriousness of the potential harm. Risk assessment is an important tool for preventing RSIs and for finding the factors that need to change in order to improve the situation for RSI sufferers. By examining what and how an individual is doing a task, it is possible to make the right adjustments.

Risk assessment is a continuous process. Here's a four-step method for assessing and controlling risks:

1.   **Identify hazards** Think about what you are doing and identify anything that could lead to RSIs. Review your workstation design and safer work practices to find out if your equipment and the way you are using it may lead to RSIs. Think about your posture and how much time you spend on your computer. Employers should ask their employees what they think the risks and hazards are in their jobs.

2. **Assess**. Decide what to do: Decide what you can do to change the hazards you have found. Prioritize the hazards, focusing on those that are most likely to cause serious harm. Then, consider if you can modify your workstation, take more breaks, change your posture, or use software or computer functions to reduce your risk of getting injured.

3. **Act**. Reduce the hazards. Make the changes you decided on. You may be able to make some of the changes right away, like using reams of paper to raise the monitor or taking more breaks.

Some of the improvements may cost money, like buying a new mouse or chair.

4. **Monitor the changes**. Pay attention to how you feel after you improve your situation. Do you feel more/less aches, pains, or stress? How comfortable are you? Do your symptoms worsen or get better? You may need to start the assessment process over again if the changes don't create the improvements you want. Record your findings.

RSI-sufferer's story: *Pat is a government employee who works in a large office. She spends much of the day on her computer. One day, she started feeling pain in her arms and neck. She asked her co-worker to help her figure out why she was having pain all of a sudden, when she hadn't had any problems in the past. Using the assessment process, they discovered that Pat's working surface was too high. They realized that when new furniture was installed throughout the office the previous week, all the work surfaces were set at the same height. As Pat is shorter than most people, her desk was too high, so she was working with her neck bent to see the monitor and her wrists bent to reach the keys. Once her desk was adjusted to the right height for her, all of Pat's symptoms disappeared.*

2) Videotape Assessment

Another way to assess the dangers of repetitive motion is to videotape a person doing the work. Videotaping is the best way to see exactly what you are doing that could cause injury. It's also a great way to see improvements after changes are made.

3) Finding and Eliminating RSI Hazards

Repetitive Strain Injury: A Computer User's Guide has a repetitive strain troubleshooting guide to help people figure out what they are doing to cause them pain. Following are the key points:

Problem	Possible Cause	Possible Remedy
Headache, neck pain	Screen too high	Lower screen
	Spectacles not right for computer work	Get new prescription
	Muscle tension	Relax, stretch
Overall neck pain	Chin jutting forward	Massage, stretch, tuck chin in
Pain on one side of neck	Monitor to the side, not in front	Move monitor in front
Pain in elbow	Table too high, overuse	Lower table, take breaks, work slower, stretch, strengthen muscles
Pain on top of forearm, little finger side	Typing with fingers flat, holding little finger up while typing, bending wrists to left or right	Keep fingernails short and wrists straight, technique retraining
Pain in fingertips	Pounding keyboard	Use light touch
Pain in thumb or thumb side of wrist	Overuse, holding thumb up while typing, hitting space	Breaks, use fingers for space bar, technique retraining

157

	bar too hard.	
Pain on bottom of forearm	Overuse, hands bent down from wrists	Breaks, stretching, massage, posture retraining
Numbness in fingers, pain in wrists	Resting wrists on edge of desk or wrist rest, edge of desk cutting into wrists	Don't rest wrists whilst typing

Chapter 16) Wrist Pain - Causes

While this book concentrates largely on Carpal Tunnel Syndrome, it is also important to look at other types of repetitive strain injuries that affect the wrist as these can sometimes cause the symptoms of CTS to develop, especially if the tendons start to swell and put pressure on the median nerve.

In all cases of RSI, it is essential that the symptoms and the causes behind it are addressed as soon as possible rather than ignoring them. If the symptoms are ignored, or if the person continues the same repetitive action, then it is likely that the condition will worsen to the point that the CTS becomes chronic (long-term) and it will be even more difficult to treat.

1) Wrist Tendonitis

Tendonitis refers to the inflammation of a tendon. It is referred to as tendinopathy these days as doctors feel that that it gives a more accurate description of what is going on in the wrist.

However, there are still differing opinions on this and some doctors will consider it tendonitis for the first 6-8 weeks, and then diagnose it as tendinopathy if the tendon fails to heal after that and it is thought that there is wear to the tendon.

Symptoms of tendonitis or tendinopathy include pain and discomfort around the wrist area. The pain will often feel like a burning pain, which is often a sure sign of inflammation.

Early treatments for tendonitis of the wrist include icing the affected area, taking anti-inflammatories and pain killers and resting the painful wrist.

Sometimes, but not always, a therapist will suggest strapping the wrist. However, if the patient has already lost mobility in the wrist as a result of their tendonitis then this is not a good idea. Strapping the wrist area will impair the mobility of the wrist further still, and when the patient begins to recover, it can be much more difficult to get the mobility back. Also, if the wrist is strapped for long periods of time, this can cause muscle wasting, leading to a further weakness that can leave people vulnerable to further injury.

Before strapping or splinting a sore wrist, speak to a physiotherapist first and they can determine if strapping the wrist is the correct course of action.

One way to gently rest the affected wrist without strapping it is to use the other arm as a "sling". Rest the affected wrist on the lower part of the opposite arm to give the inflamed wrist some cushioning and support, but only do this if it is comfortable to do so and not for long periods of time.

A massage is a good way to reduce the tension and tightness that will have accumulated in the wrist area due to the overuse of the tendons or muscles.

Massage should be carried out by an expert in order to be effective and should concentrate on the wrist, hand, forearm and shoulder area.

2) Rotator Cuff Tendinopathy

Rotator cuff tendinopathy is a painful shoulder condition that is often the result of repetitive actions. It is not uncommon to develop shoulder pain when a patient has Carpal Tunnel Syndrome or another overuse injury in the lower part of the arm.

If the wrist has become weakened due to the CTS, this will mean the muscles further up the arm will have to compensate, and this will often mean that the shoulder - specifically the rotator cuff muscle – will have to work much harder, thus overworking the tendons in the shoulder.

Rotator Cuff Tendinopathy can be extremely debilitating, limiting the ability to reach clothes in wardrobes, do up buttons or even tie up shoe laces, so if you experience any type of shoulder pain don't just hope that it will go away – get it looked at. In addition, if you are also suffering from RSI or Carpal Tunnel Syndrome, explain this to your specialist or your physio so that they are aware that there is a weakness lower down in the arm that is contributing to the problem.

In most cases of tendinopathy, the doctor will advise resting the shoulder, and depending on how severe the pain is, you might not have any other choice in the matter other than resting the shoulder.

Anti-inflammatories will be prescribed in the early stages along with painkillers if the pain is severe.

Patients will often be referred to a physiotherapist to get a personalised exercise programme. They might also be referred to a hand specialist; they will help the patient to address the working position of the hands and give advice on wrist strengthening exercises if the patient has a weakness there.

If there is a weakness in the wrist, it is likely that splints will also be prescribed to give the hands some support while taking the stress away from the shoulder area.

3) Writer's Cramp

Writer's Cramp is also referred to as Dystonia. It is caused when the muscles contract and go into spasm.

The symptoms of this condition are usually noticeable when performing certain tasks, such as gripping a pen or pencil.

There are a limited amount of treatments for this condition. Botox injections to relax the spasms and medications are among the most common therapies.

4) Bursitis of the Wrist

Bursitis of the wrist occurs when the bursa sac becomes inflamed. This often happens when a patients has been carrying out repetitive actions that cause friction and inflammation.

Symptoms of bursitis include swelling in the wrist area, stiffness in the wrist joint, pain when typing and the wrist might feel hot, which is a sign of inflammation.

Treatments of bursitis are pretty much the same as they are for tendonitis; heat and warmth therapy, anti-inflammatory medication such as ibuprofen and naproxen, rest, and ultrasound treatments to help to reduce pain and swelling.

5) Sprain

A sprain occurs when the ligaments of the wrist become damaged, usually as the result of a fall. Symptoms of a sprain include swelling, pain and problems moving the wrist.

The best approach to healing a sprain is to rest the affected area and take medication to help deal with the pain and inflammation. The wrist can also be rested in a support while it recovers or put in a crepe bandage, but not if this limits the mobility of the wrist.

These types of injuries can take six to eight weeks before they are completely healed.

6) Strain

A strain affects the muscles as opposed to the ligaments and a strain occurs when the muscles have been stretched or torn. In the case of a strain, the joint should be immobilised to protect it from further damage and advice should be sought from a doctor if the pain continues or gets worse.

Treatment will usually consist of painkillers and rest. Again, typical healing times for a strain can be up to eight weeks, but will vary on the person and the severity of the strain.

7) Arthritis

Arthritis is a common cause of wrist pain and this can also increase the likelihood of developing Carpal Tunnel Syndrome due to the swelling and inflammation that can put pressure on the median nerve.

Symptoms of arthritis include pain and swelling and a loss of movement in the wrist area.

Arthritis is generally treated with anti-inflammatory medication, cortisone injections and splinting. Exercises should also be prescribed in order to maintain movement in the joint and to prevent muscle loss.

In severe cases, a joint fusion or a joint reconstruction might need to be considered.

8) Tenosynovitis

Tenosynovitis is an inflammation of the tendon sheath. Repetitive actions can often contribute to the development of this condition so actions like typing can cause it.

Symptoms include pain on movement and swelling. The area may also feel hot.

Treatment will include rest, anti-inflammatory medication and icing the joint to reduce swelling.

RSI-sufferers story: *"I don't actually know how I coped - I just did. My husband had to do many extra chores - I couldn't chop vegetables, I would drop things and break many jars/plates/glasses in the kitchen, turning keys in locks was impossible with my right hand - as was general things like doing up bra straps, washing and drying my hair."* Source: Watson, M. 2009. Investigating the experiences of people with RSI. http://etheses.qmu.ac.uk/133/

9) Fracture

Fractures are more often than not the result of a fall and can sometimes be mistaken for a sprain or a strain.

There may be bruising and swelling around the wrist area, and the joint may appear deformed if the fracture is severe.

Surgery is often required to repair a fracture; however, just casting the joint might also be effective if the fracture isn't too bad.

Any patient experiencing severe pain after a fall should get an x-ray to rule out a fracture.

Chapter 17) Other Types of Lower Body Pain

1) Cubital Tunnel Syndrome

Cubital Tunnel Syndrome is another form of nerve entrapment that affects the nerves. In this condition, the ulna nerve is affected as opposed to the median nerve that becomes entrapped in cases of Carpal Tunnel Syndrome. The condition is sometimes referred to as Ulna nerve neuritis.

It develops when the nerve in the elbow becomes entrapped. Pain and tingling in the fingers, specifically the in the ring finger or little finger, are one of the main symptoms of Cubital Tunnel Syndrome.

As the condition progresses, patients might find that they begin to lose sensation in their hand and everyday tasks such as gripping things may become difficult. In Cubital Tunnel Syndrome, patients are also prone to developing muscle weakness.

There are several factors that can contribute to this type of nerve entrapment and these include an underlying health condition such as diabetes or arthritis, an injury or trauma to the area, or a poor sleeping posture. It can also be common among people who carry out a lot of repetitive activity.

a) Diagnosis of Cubital Tunnel Syndrome

This condition is diagnosed by carrying out nerve conduction studies to find out how well the electrical nerve impulses are firing. These tests will also give the neurologist an idea of where the entrapment is in the ulna nerve.

b) Treatment of Cubital Tunnel Syndrome

Often, surgery is not required to treat this condition, unless the symptoms have become severe. In cases of Cubital Tunnel Syndrome, conservative measures are favoured first. Your consultant might suggest wearing an elbow pad to give the area some protection and medication such as anti-inflammatory medicines might be prescribed.

Ice might also be suggested to help relieve any swelling or inflammation.

c) Surgery

Surgery for Cubital Tunnel Syndrome will involve decompressing the affected nerve. The surgery is carried out under a general anaesthetic and is usually a day case so there should be no need for an extended hospital stay.

The affected arm will be placed in a sling after the surgery and it will be up to six weeks before this can be removed. Patients might also be given exercises to do to aid their recovery.

Once the dressing has been removed, a physio will work with the patient to help them regain the strength and mobility that they have lost during their recuperation period.

The recovery time for surgery can take up to a year and the patient will need to take care that they don't do any activity that might aggravate the nerve such as overusing the affected arm.

2) Medial epicondylitis

The humerous – commonly known as the funny bone – contains medial epicondyle. In cases of medial epicondylitis, these get inflamed. This is often referred to as Golfer's Elbow.

However, it isn't just limited to Golfers. Anyone who participates in repetitive activity such as typing, playing computer games, texting, playing a musical instrument or digging in the garden can find themselves vulnerable to this type of inflammation.

Medial Epicondylitis Treatment

The treatment for Golfer's Elbow is the same for other forms of tendon overuse and inflammation. Ice packs can be useful to reduce swelling and ease some of the burning pain that is associated with inflammatory conditions.

Patients will be advised to rest the affected area. A doctor will also prescribe anti-inflammatory medication or suggest steroid injections if the pain is severe and the inflammation doesn't subside.

It might also be advised that the patient wears a splint to protect their elbow from overuse; using ice can help to relieve some of the inflammation.

When applying ice, do not place it directly on the skin as it may cause burns or chilblains. Instead, wrap the ice pack in a towel. It is also advisable to not use ice in the same area for more than 10-20 minutes.

3) Elbow Bursitis

Bursitis can occur in the elbow joint, causing pain in the elbow region. This happens when the bursa sac gets inflamed and can be caused by repetitive activity and sometimes by a sudden impact to the elbow joint.

In response to repetitive stress or sudden injury, the bursa will swell and become inflamed. There might also be fluid in the bursa sac, which will contribute to the pain and swelling.

Treatments for Elbow Bursitis

Since overuse is the most common cause of this painful condition, rest is the best solution. If you are unable to rest, for instance if you can't take time off work, or if you are a student doing a lot of computer or written work, then the best option is to make a few modifications to the work area.

First of all, make sure that the elbow isn't rested directly on the desk when you work. Get an elbow rest with a gel cushioning so that you can rest your elbow without putting too much pressure on it.

If it is a minor case, there might not be any need for medication, but if the symptoms are bad enough to need to see a doctor, they are likely to prescribe anti-inflammatories.

Placing ice around the elbow can also reduce pain and swelling.

If fluid has gathered in the bursa sac then medical intervention might be required to drain the excess fluid, especially if it is causing pain.

Patients with this condition can sometimes go on to develop an infection in this area so look out for any symptoms of infection such as an increased amount of pain or redness in the affected elbow.

This is a condition that often clears up on its own over time, and doesn't normally require surgery, except in severe cases.

4) Elbow Tendonitis

Elbow tendonitis is a common repetitive strain injury. Again, typing, texting or playing computer games are all common causes of this condition, but playing sports such as darts, tennis or golf can also cause it.

Tendonitis can be extremely painful and it can restrict the movement of the arm when it occurs in the elbow joint.

Treatment for elbow tendonitis

Resting the arm is the only real option as the elbow needs to be rested from the activity that has caused it. As with elbow bursitis, if complete rest isn't possible you'll need to alter your work habits.

Make sure that the elbow isn't rested directly against the desk and wear an elbow rest to give the joint some support while it heals. Anti-inflammatories are likely to be prescribed to help ease the pain and ice will reduce swelling.

Cases of elbow tendonitis can take 6-8 weeks to heal and longer if the elbow continues to be under repetitive stress as it won't get a chance to heal.

5) Cervical Spondylosis

This type of arthritis is quite common as people grow older. When the joints of the spine get worn, they can cause nerves to become entrapped, causing shooting and tingling pains down the arm and in the elbow.

Treatment for Cervical Spondylosis

Treatment usually involves the prescription of pain medication. Posture is also important to ensure that the patient isn't putting an undue pressure on their spine.

Sleeping positions will also need to be adjusted to ensure that the neck and spine are properly supported at night.

Exercises might also be prescribed by a physiotherapist and neck stretches can be helpful.

6) Frozen Shoulder

A frozen shoulder is an extremely debilitating condition and can leave the simplest thing such as putting on clothes almost impossible.

When a patient has a frozen shoulder, this means that that the connective tissue around the glenohumeral joint has become inflamed. The inflammation will cause a limitation in the movements of the shoulder and the condition can be chronic. Symptoms often come on without any warning and in some cases they will disappear without warning as well.

Patients with diabetes or with thyroid problems can be more prone to this condition.

Treatment for Frozen Shoulder

Typical treatments include pain medication and physical therapy. An occupational therapist will help the patient to find effective methods of managing household tasks and chores.

Surgery will be considered in the most serious of cases, however, the condition might just go away on its own.

Chapter 18) Gadgets for Carpal Tunnel Syndrome

In the advanced stages of Carpal Tunnel Syndrome many patients develop problems with the strength in their wrists or hands. This can make managing everyday tasks extremely challenging but there are many gadgets that can help to make life around the home a little easier.

Firstly, speak to an Occupational Therapist. They are the best person to advise you on the kind of items that are available to help around the home. Often, some of these gadgets are available on the NHS; however, if they cannot be obtained this way, many of the items are reasonably priced to buy.

1) Gripping

A loss of strength in the hand or wrist can lead to problems such as difficulty in undoing jars or bottles. There are, however, many helpful gadgets to help with this problem.

Jar grippers can take the stress out of the wrist when opening jars, one touch can openers or squeeze can openers are useful for anyone with wrist pain that can't turn a tin opener, and there are tools for opening bottle caps, ring pulls and bottle tops. These gadgets aren't just useful for people with Carpal Tunnel Syndrome, but they also help to reduce wrist pain.

2) Grip Strengtheners

There are many hand-held pieces of equipment that have been designed to help develop grip strength. It is a good idea to use this equipment as soon as you notice any loss of muscle strength as it might help to arrest it, however, you will need to be careful not to overuse the muscles and tendons or there's a chance of making the symptoms of Carpal Tunnel worse.

There is a range of equipment to choose from, the most popular items are adjustable grip strengtheners, resistance hand exercisers, adjustable tension exercisers or hand and finger exercisers.

When choosing this type of exercise equipment, choose something that has a comfortable, easy to grip handle so it doesn't cause discomfort when performing the exercises.

Only do as many repetitions as is comfortable and warm your hands up before performing any exercises by circling the hands to loosen up the wrists, and follow the stretch exercises for the wrists that are detailed earlier in the book after you have completed the strength work.

3) Writing

If writing has become difficult then there are aids that will act as a holder for a pen or pencil and make gripping much easier. These tools are helpful for patients with arthritis and Carpal Tunnel Syndrome.

There are many different makes available; Aidapt and Ability are just two of the manufacturers that have these products.

4) Eating

A range of cutlery and cups are available for people with nerve conditions such as Carpal Tunnel Syndrome and for Arthritis. These come with extra-large handles that allow a comfortable grip and they are adjustable so that they can be adapted according to your needs.

There are several brands of these available and they are easy to obtain online.

5) Kitchen Ware

Preparing meals can become quite a challenge for patients if they have lost the ability to be able to grip properly. However, there are plenty of products that are now available to help a patient maintain their independence.

An occupational therapist can offer advice on the safest ways to prepare foods and they can visit a patient in their own home to give advice on preparing meals and gadgets that will be helpful. It is important that a patient does seek advice before purchasing this type of equipment as they need to know that it is right for them.

For patients that are unable to access occupational therapy services through their GP or consultant, the best way is to contact your local Social Services department at the council. They will often have a form that can be filled out online and the patient can request a visit.

Grants are also available if adaptions need to be made to make the kitchen safer.

6) Jar Openers and Bottle Openers

Many manufacturers now have products available to make opening jars and bottles easy; these products aid with gripping, which makes handling everyday tasks more manageable.

7) Compression Support Gloves

These gloves are a useful "gadget" for patients suffering from arthritis. The gloves have been designed with patients with arthritis in mind, and not for patients with Carpal Tunnel Syndrome, so if you are thinking of buying this product then seek advice first to check that they are right for your needs.

The gloves provide additional support to the hands, giving extra strength to help the grip. They also provide extra warmth to the hand and the wrists and apply gentle compression to the area.

They are designed to relieve pain and increase circulation; they are a useful tool for patients that aren't as nimble fingered as they once were and for patients that want to continue with hobbies, as they will help to maintain dexterity.

8) Hobbies

Whatever your hobby is, there is no reason why it should be limited due to Carpal Tunnel Syndrome. Obviously, you shouldn't do anything that only serves to make the pain worse, but hobbies such as crafts and gardening can still be carried out by buying tools that have been designed to make these past times more manageable.

Chapter 19) Rights and Responsibilities in the Workplace

1) Duties on Employers

Employers must follow safety and health regulations. They have a general responsibility to ensure the safety and health of work and take reasonable measures to control risks. They must:

- Appoint a competent person to help meet their health and safety responsibilities.

- Write a health and safety policy for the business.

- Assess the risks.

- Work with health and safety representatives to protect employees.

- Display the HSE-approved health and safety law poster or give each worker the leaflet equivalent to the poster.

- Tell employees about the risks in language they can understand.

- Provide health and safety training.

- Provide any equipment and protective clothing their employees need, at no charge to the employees.

- Provide toilets, washing facilities and safe drinking water.

- Provide adequate first aid supplies, including, at a minimum: a stocked first-aid box and a person appointed to take charge of first aid. Employers must inform all employees about the first aid system they have in place;

175

- Have insurance that covers employees who get ill or hurt from work and display a copy (electronic or hard copy) of the insurance certificate where workers can easily read it.

- Keep an accident book if you have 10 or more employees (required under social security law).

- Coordinate with other contractors or employers that share the workplace or provide agency workers to protect the health and safety of everyone.

- Report major injuries and deaths at work to the HSE Incident Contact Centre at 0845 300 9923.

- Report other injuries, illnesses, and dangerous incidents at www.hse.gov.uk.

2) Rights and Responsibilities of Employees

Employees have the right to work in environments where health and safety risks are properly controlled. Employers are responsible for controlling those work-related health and safety risks, as discussed above.

Workers have the right to be provided with safety equipment free of charge. As a worker you can stop work and leave your work area without being disciplined if you have reasonable concerns about your safety. You have the right to have rest breaks during the day, time off from work during the work week, and an annual paid holiday.

Workers who are unable to work because of work-related RSIs may qualify for Industrial Injuries Disablement Benefits (IIDB). Benefits are paid whether or not the person is still working. The amount of the benefit is based on the age of the employee and the severity and longevity of the injury or illness. Directgov (http://www.direct.gov.uk) has more information on IIDB and how to apply for benefits.

Workers also have the right to make injury claims against their employers if they believe their repetitive strain injuries resulted from their jobs.

- In 2002, a court ordered Barclays Bank to pay £244,000 to a former employee who had to give up work at the age of 28 because of pain in her right hand. [The worker] had worked as a bank clerk, and argued that a defective workstation caused her to perform keyboard work in an unsuitable posture. Her symptoms developed over two years, after which time [she] was unable to tie her shoes or even comb her hair.

- A personal assistant was awarded £40,062 for work-related bilateral (both hands) carpal tunnel syndrome and cervical spondylosis. The personal assistant spent 80 percent of her time typing documents with inadequate breaks in order to meet tight deadlines. Plus, the position of her computer monitor required her to turn her head at a 45-degree angle, making her RSIs worse. The court ruled that the employer was in breach of statutory duty by failing to enforce breaks and control the high workload. Claims Management Company www.antriumlegal.com

As a worker you have the right to tell your employer about your safety and health concerns. HSE encourages workers to talk with their supervisors, managers, or safety representatives if they have concerns about their safety work. If that doesn't resolve the problem, you can contact the Environmental Health Department at your local council if you work in an office, shop, restaurant, place of worship, pub, club, nursery, playground, or hotel. If you work for other premises or government offices you should contact the local office of the Health and Safety Executive, which can be found in the telephone book or at http://www.hse.gov.uk/contact/maps/index.htm. It's your right to contact HSE or your local authority if your employer doesn't help you with your safety concerns; your employer is not allowed to discipline you for contacting them.

Workers have health and safety responsibilities too. They must help their employers control risks by:

- Following safety training.

- Paying attention to their own and co-workers' health and safety.

- Cooperating with employers' health and safety programmes.

- Reporting suspected work hazards to the employer, supervisor, or safety representative as soon as possible.

- Reporting injuries as soon as possible.

3) Returning to Work

The good news is that the majority of workers who get RSIs and CTS will be able to return to work. It may take a while for them to return, and they may need accommodations to do their jobs, but it is to everyone's advantage to help employees return as soon as possible. Workers who are off the job for extended periods of time may suffer depression, isolation, financial insecurity, and difficulty with relationships. The fact is that the longer a worker stays off the job due to injury, illness, or disability, the less likely he or she is ever to return to work.

Returning to work is not as simple as it may sound. There's no one-size-fits-all approach; each worker presents a unique situation requiring individual attention. Employers whose employees do repetitive work should have return-to-work systems in place before anyone gets hurt. Employers should tell their employees that it is company policy to help them return to work after an injury or illness. They should also monitor and record all sickness absences, whether work-related or not. The data collected from monitoring and recording can be used to identify trends and problems in the workplace and correct them to avoid further injuries or illnesses. The Chartered Institute of Personnel and Development (CIPD) offers a free online toolkit to help employers management absences (http://www.cipd.co.uk/hr-resources/practical-tools/absence-management.aspx).

The Statement of Fitness for Work, or fit note, plays an important role in returning to work. From 6 April 2010, the fit note replaces the sick note, or Medical Statement. When a person is unable to work for more than seven days, the doctor writes a fit note, which advises the employer if the employee is "not fit to work," "fit for work" or "may be fit for work."

An employee who "may be fit for work" may be able to return to the job if the employer provides the necessary support. Employer and employee need to work together to implement the suggestions of the doctor. In the fit note the doctor gives information about how the condition will affect the work the employee can do. The doctor may recommend:

- Phased return to work. Gradual increase in work hours, days, or duties;

- Change in work hours. Flexibility to start and/or leave work earlier or later;

- Changes to work duties. For example, more time face-to-face with customers to reduce time on the computer; and/or

- Adaptations to the workplace. For example, providing alternative computer equipment.

If an employer is unable to make the changes an employee needs in order to return to work, the employee cannot return until he or she has recovered more fully. It behoves employers to help employees return to work as quickly as medically advisable. It's better for the business and better for the worker.

RSI-sufferer's story: *"I still can't write, cook, push a pram, kayak or a thousand other things but I work full-time (with the help of an understanding employer and voice-activated software-*

which I am using at the moment). I can also at least play (to some extent) with my children, feed them, and offer some help with childcare. I still have off days, frequently suffer pain but have improved so much." Source: Watson, M. 2009. Investigating the experiences of people with RSI. http://etheses.qmu.ac.uk/133/

4) Ergonomic Management Programme

"Ergonomics is the scientific discipline concerned with the understanding of the interactions among humans and other elements of a system . . . that applies theory principles, data and methods to design in order to optimize human well-being . . . ergonomists contribute to design and evaluation of tasks, jobs, products, environments and systems in order to make them compatible with the needs, abilities, and limitations of people."— International Ergonomics Association

Ergonomics means fitting the workplace to the worker by modifying or redesigning the job, workstation, tool, or environment. Ergonomics draws from the fields of engineering, and medical and health sciences to optimize the work environment. By identifying ergonomic hazards that can result in an injury or illness, and correcting these hazards, employees can be provided a healthier workplace" Source : www.safety.com

It is much harder to change people than to change furniture, tools and work practices. Ergonomics is a very important concept for reducing work-related RSIs.

The more employees are involved in the ergonomic process, the more successful the process will be. This makes sense because workers are the experts about their jobs; they know more about the hazards and how to correct them than anyone else. Together with managers, supervisors, and health and safety professionals, workers solve problems and take charge of injury prevention.

The United States Occupational Safety and Health Administration, or OSHA, has established guidelines for protecting workers from ergonomic hazards that result in injuries to the musculoskeletal system, including RSIs and other conditions. Whilst each workplace needs to establish its own RSI-prevention programme, the OSHA guidelines provide a framework for those efforts. The following 7-step process is based on OSHA's guidelines:

a) Provide Management Support

Maintaining a safe and healthful workplace where risks are eliminated (or at least reasonably reduced) requires the strong and visible support of top management. Management needs to allocate sufficient resources (finances and personnel). OSHA recommends that employers develop clear goals, assign responsibilities to achieve those goals, provide necessary resources and make sure the designated employees fulfil their responsibilities.

b) Involve Employees

Employees know the most about their jobs and the hazards of their jobs. Ergonomic programmes are much more likely to succeed when employees are involved in significant ways. Employees should be encouraged to voice their concerns and ideas; discuss work methods; participate in the design of work, equipment, procedures, and training; evaluate equipment; and participate in ergonomics task groups.

c) Identify Problems

Organisations need systematic ways to identify hazards. Methods may include reviewing injury and illness records, investigation reports, and insurance claims; interviewing, observing, and surveying employees; conducting risk assessments; and observing workplace conditions.

d) Implement Solutions

Once the problems are known, appropriate solutions can be developed and implemented. Solutions typically involve changes in equipment and/or changes in how the work is done (work practices).

e) Address Reports of Injuries

Management needs to respond promptly to injury reports, making sure employees receive appropriate treatment and follow up, including return-to-work programs. Injury reports and logs can help identify any ongoing problems.

f) Provide Training

Training in ergonomics will make employees, managers and supervisors more effective participants in the ergonomic process ad programme. They also need training in the RSI hazards of the workplace, how to identify them, and what to do in response. Early reporting of symptoms and hazards should be part of training. Studies show that as many as 90 percent of workers do not receive training on RSI risks, symptoms, and safe working procedures.

g) Evaluate Effectiveness of Ergonomic Programme

After the changes have been made, workplaces need to find out whether or not the changes have been effective in eliminating or at least reducing the RSI or CTS hazards. Any remaining problems can be dealt with as part of the evaluation.

RSI-sufferer's story: *When editors at a major U.S. newspaper complained about outdated and uncomfortable office equipment, the purchasing manager took the complaints seriously. To make sure the new furniture would make the improvements the editors wanted, the purchasing manger selected employees from every department to try out new equipment. Based on the employees' choices, the purchasing manager bought equipment for employees to test. Chairs were bought first, then keyboard trays, then desks.*

After the testers had time to "live with" the trial equipment for a reasonable amount of time, the purchasing manager purchased new equipment for all departments based on the testers' recommendations. Source: HSE

5) Safety in a Weak Economy

When the economy is sluggish, employers often look to their safety and health programmes for cutting costs. Most employers find that cutting back on safety to save money comes back to haunt them in the long run. By slashing safety budgets companies risk expensive work injuries and the bad publicity, low morale and production losses that accompany them. They also risk losing other valued workers, because highly skilled workers will look for other jobs if they perceive that their employer are not paying adequate attention to safety. By maintaining a safe working environment companies remain prepared for the eventual economic recovery.

Workers are also endangered by layoffs. With fewer workers on the job each one may be expected to do more work or to work faster. They also may be assigned to jobs for which they are not fully trained or experienced. The heavier workload, faster pace and lack of training are all risk factors for RSIs.

6) Stress on the Job

Improving workstations and work practices addresses the physical hazards of job. That's important, but it's only part of the solution for reducing RSIs. The other part is harder to look at and, perhaps, harder to change. We're talking about the psychosocial aspects of the work environment. "Psychosocial" refers to interactions between people—how well people communicate, get along and support each other. Psychosocial hazards are elements of the workplace--such as management, organisation and environment--that can contribute to physical or psychological harm. A workplace can have the most up-to-date ergonomic equipment and training, but if it doesn't feel good to work there, workers are likely to get hurt. True ergonomics deal with all the factors that make up a workplace physical and psychosocial.

"Psychosocial" and "stress" are two words that often go together. The National Institute for Occupational Safety and Health, or NIOSH, defines workplace stress as: "...the harmful physical and emotional responses that occur when the requirements of the job do not match the capabilities, resources, or needs of the worker. Job stress can lead to poor health and even injury." According to NIOSH workplace stress can cause or aggravate a number of health problems, including musculoskeletal disorders.

There's no doubt that job stress is on the rise worldwide. A survey conducted for the European Agency for Safety and Health at Work (EU-OSHA),found that job-related stress is a concern for the large majority of the European workforce. Seventy-nine percent of the managers surveyed think stress is as important an issue for their companies as accidents.

Stress sets off a "fight or flight" reaction in the brain: the pulse quickens, breathing deepens, and muscles tense up. When the stress resolves, the brain goes back to normal and all is well, but when stress is constant, the body remains in its heightened state, causing undo wear and tear on the body's systems and tissues. Plus, stress is also distracting; it's hard to focus on doing your job safely when you are all wound up.

a) Job Stressors
It's no secret what makes a job stressful:
- High work demand, including long work hours/mandatory overtime
- Tight deadlines
- Shift work
- Lack of family friendly policies
- Bad relationship with supervisor

- Racist, sexists, or bullying supervisor
- Unsafe or unpleasant working conditions, including ergonomic problems
- Lack of co-worker support
- Work that is either too challenging or not challenging enough
- Not being appreciated for your work
- Lack of control over work
- No possibilities for advancement within the organisation
- Dissatisfaction with the job
- Ambiguity about job responsibilities
- Too much or too little responsibility
- Poor communication within the organisation
- Concern about job security from plant closings/layoff/relocation/automation

A stress and musculoskeletal disorder study by HSE found that high exposure to physical and psychosocial risk factors on the job increased the likelihood of reporting musculoskeletal complaints, including neck, should, elbow/forearm, hand/wrist, and back complaints.

b) Reducing Stress

What can be done about job stress? NIOSH finds that recognition of employees for good work performance, opportunities for career development, organisational culture that values individual workers, and management actions that are consistent with the values of the organisation are associated with low-stress and high-productivity workplaces.

Solutions vary with each workplace, and might include:

-       Ensuring that the workload is in line with the employees' abilities.

- Designing jobs that are rewarding and allow workers to use their skills.
- Clearly defining roles and responsibilities.
- Involving employees in decisions that affect their jobs.
- Improving communications.
- Providing opportunities for social interaction amongst employees.
- Establishing flexible work schedules that support employees in meeting their family and personal responsibilities.

Personal factors also play a role in the individual's ability to manage stress. In other words, some people are better able to handle stress than others. For people who turn pressure into stress, decision-making, efficiency and compliance with safety practices can be compromised. So, in addition to making changes in work equipment and physical environment, employers can help reduce stress on the job by providing training on stress management.

c) HSE Management Standards

HSE has developed Management Standards for work-related stress that establishes a process for controlling stress and identifying the characteristics of an organisation where stress is being managed effectively. The approach involves five steps:

1. Identify the risk factors.
2. Determine who can be harmed and how.
3. Evaluate the risks.
4. Record your findings.
5. Monitor and review.

The Management Standards address six key areas:

1. Demand. Workload, work pattern, work environment.
2. Control. What workers have to say about the way they do their work.
3. Support. The encouragement and resources provided by the employer, managers, and colleagues.
4. Relationships. Promoting positive working to avoid conflicts. Dealing with unacceptable behaviour.
5. Role. Whether workers understand their roles and whether the organisation ensures workers do not have conflicting roles.
6. Change. How change is managed and communicated in the organisation.

Experts agree that changes to major areas such as these require the participation of everyone involved. It's not enough to marginally involve employees in the solution. As NIOSH puts it: *"Bringing workers and managers together in a committee or problem-solving group may be an especially useful approach for developing a stress prevention program. Research has shown these participatory efforts to be effective in dealing with ergonomic problems in the workplace, partly because they capitalize on workers' firsthand knowledge of hazards encountered in their jobs."*

The more employees participate in identifying stress reduction needs and developing prevention programs, the more specific the solutions will be for that workplace. The combination of employee engagement and success in reducing stress in the work environment is key to reducing the risks for RSIs.

Chapter 20) Relevant Regulations

Many countries have regulations governing the use of computers in the workplace. It is impossible to list the regulations for all countries; so following are key regulations from the UK and the USA. In addition to national regulations, localities may have their own rules for safe computer use. Laws and regulations change all the time so the information below is correct at the time of print but might change.

1) Great Britain

a) Health and Safety at Work Act (HASAW)

Primary regulation concerning occupational safety and health in the UK. Employers must assess risks to their employees and other people who might be affected by what they do, such as children or the public. They must take reasonable steps to minimise the risks. In addition, employers must protect employees after they return to work if they are more vulnerable to risks because of injury, illness, or disability.

b) Workplace (Health, Safety, & Welfare) Regulations

Applies to most workplaces (except those involving construction works on construction sites, in or on ships, or below ground at a mine) and covers a number of basic health, safety, and welfare issues.

c) Health and Safety (Display Screen Equipment) Rules

Employers who have employees who habitually use display screen equipment (DSE) as a significant part of their normal work must:

- Analyse workstations to assess and reduce risks. Employers must look at the whole workstation, including equipment, furniture, and the work environment. They must also look at the task being done and any special needs of the individual employee. Employers should assess workstations when a new workstation is set up, when a new user starts work, or when a major change is made to an existing workstation or to the use of the workstation.

- Ensure workstations meet specified minimum requirements covering chairs, lighting, screens, keyboards, desks, software, and the work environment.

- Plan work activities to include breaks or changes of activity depending on the nature of the activity. The law does not specify the number or length of breaks.

- Provide eye and eyesight tests on request by employees who habitually use DSE as a significant part of their normal day-to-day work. The employer must pay for spectacles if special corrective spectacles are required for DSE work. The employer does not have to pay for normal spectacles.

- Provide health and safety information and training on how to use their workstations safely to avoid health problems. The employer must also provide information on computer use health and safety and on what the employer is doing to comply with the regulation. Topics should include posture, adjusting furniture, desk organisation, adjusting screens and lighting to avoid reflections and glare, breaks and changes of activity, risk assessments, how to apply for an eye test and how to report problems about their work.

An IT Assessments Officer was awarded £2,750 in injury compensation for having developed tenosynovitis in the right wrist at work. The employer conceded it had breached sections of the Health and Safety (Display Screen Equipment) Regulations.

d) Disability Discrimination Act (DDA)

Employers must make reasonable adjustments to disabled employees' work to make sure they are not treated less favourably than other employees.

e) Reporting Regulations

Under the Reporting of Injuries, Diseases and Dangerous Occurrences Regulations (RIDDOR), employers, the self-employed and people in control of work premises are required to report serious workplace accidents, occupational diseases and close calls. RSIs are reportable if they lead to a major injury or result in absence lasting more than three working days.

f) Employee Rights Act

Employers must adopt fair procedures before dismissing an employee for being absent from work due to sickness.

g) Provision and Use of Work Equipment Regulations

Employers must assess and prevent or control health and safety risks from equipment they use at work.

h) Data Protection Act

Employers must keep certain sickness absence data.

i) Management of Health & Safety at Work Regulations

Employers must assess risks that arise from work activities, including people who are not in their employment but may be affected by the work. Affected people may include children who are affected by work at their school, the general public or others.

j) Employment Act (Dispute Resolution)

Employers must adopt minimum discipline, dismissal, and grievance procedures.

k) Employers Liability (Compulsory Insurance) Act

Most UK employers are required to purchase Employers Liability Insurance, which covers injuries, illnesses, harassment, bullying, discrimination, unfair dismissal, work-related stress and workplace violence. It is up to the employee to show that the employer has a legal obligation to provide compensation.

2) United States

a) Occupational Safety and Health Act of 1974

Under the Occupational Safety and Health Act of 1974 (OSH Act), employers must provide employees with work and places of work that are free from recognized hazards that could cause serious harm. This is called the General Duty Clause.

Whilst some states have adopted ergonomics regulations, there is no ergonomics law for the entire country. The Occupational Safety and Health Administration (OSHA) has issued voluntary ergonomics guidelines. In the absence of a specific regulation, OSHA uses the General Duty Clause to cite and fine employers who risk ergonomic injuries to employees. OSHA has been issuing citations for ergonomic hazards since 2003.

b) Fair Labour Standards Act (FLSA)

Amongst other provisions, FLSA sets minimum standards for youth employment, addressing the hours teens can work and the type of work they can do. Many states have more stringent child labour laws as well as laws requiring breaks.

c) Workers' Compensation Laws

Most employers in the United States are required to purchase workers' compensation insurance, which pays medical costs and indemnity for employees who are injured or made ill on the job. All states have workers' compensation laws, which are administered by the states and differ from state to state. Workers' compensation insurance protects employers from legal action by employees who have been injured or made ill as a result of their work.

d) Whistleblower Protections

Whistleblower protection laws protect people (including workers) who report unsafe working conditions. In 2012, the U.S. Department of Labour fined a railroad more than $300,000 for firing an employee for reporting a work-related injury.

e) Americans with Disabilities Act (ADA)

Prohibits discrimination on the basis of employment, State and local government, public accommodations, commercial facilities, transportation and telecommunications.

Claims Management Company www.antriumlegal.com

Chapter 21) Putting it all together

1) Self Care

No matter what types of treatments you pursue, you will need to add a big dose of self-care to your CTS recovery programme. Doctors and therapists will provide information, support, therapies and assistance, but you will have to follow through. Recovery from RSI requires life changes, which **ONLY YOU** can make.

To give your body the best chance of recovery, pay attention to your overall health and wellbeing. If you feel pain or discomfort whilst performing a certain task or activity, stop immediately and take a break. Be sure to give the affected area plenty of rest. Avoid activities that make symptoms worse. Many RSI-sufferers report feeling so much better after taking a walk, no matter how long or how vigorous the walk is.

Most important of all, be kind to yourself. CTS does not make you a bad or lazy person. You are the same person you were before you became injured. Have sympathy for yourself, but don't wallow in self-pity. It's a challenging but important balance: have empathy for your situation but don't feel like a victim.

Analyse if you can do things differently e.g.

- instead of sending an email, use the phone

- instead of sending a message, get out of your chair and go and speak to the person.

- Stop playing solitaire on your laptop or PC and get yourself an old fashioned set of playing cards, much more fun and much more sociable!

- Stop chatting on Facebook and arrange to meet up somewhere so you can do the chatting whilst socialising.

- Stop surfing the web and get information the old fashioned way: from the library, magazines or from books.

To summarise: try and eliminate the time you spend using your laptop or PC.

The most important thing is to realise what exactly gives you pain and reduce the time you are doing that activity. Stop the motions that caused the injury in the first place.

You absolutely MUST take plenty of breaks from doing the same thing.

You absolutely MUST do some gentle exercises rather than sitting on your bed or in front of your laptop all day long.

You absolutely must sit in the correct posture when using a laptop or a PC.

Throughout the book there are many practical tips to help manage pain, create an ergonomic friendly workplace, finding natural therapies and helpful vitamins and minerals.

This chapter will summarise some of the most important aspects so the reader can access the information they need at a glance and how to apply it.

The main symptoms of Carpal Tunnel Syndrome are:

- Pain

- Numbness and tingling

- Weakness in the hands and wrists

2) Pain Control

The numbness and tingling felt in the hands is a sign of nerve entrapment. These symptoms can be distressing for many and finding the right method of pain control is vital.

Nerve pain is different to other types of pain and medications such as anti-inflammatories and paracetamol aren't effective for this type of discomfort.

Although anti-inflammatories might be effective at reducing pain if there is inflammation present, they won't help control nerve pain, however, NSAIDS are still often the first medication to be prescribed when a patient presents with the symptoms of Carpal Tunnel Syndrome.

If you are experiencing tingling in your fingers, then ask your doctor about the possibility of being prescribed a drug that is specifically for the nerve pain and not one just aimed at controlling inflammation.

Some forms of anti-depressant drugs and anti-seizure medication can be extremely effective at controlling this kind of nerve pain.

3) Alternative pain relief

Many people choose not to take pain medication and prefer instead to find alternatives. Supplements such as evening primrose oil and fish oil can help to reduce inflammation and ginger is also a powerful anti-inflammatory that can be bought in the form of capsules, used as a cream or bought as an essential oil. However, natural anti-inflammatories should not be taken without speaking to a GP first.

For symptoms such as tingling sensations in the fingers, supplements such as magnesium and vitamin B12 can be beneficial.

4) Weakness

Patients with advanced symptoms of Carpal Tunnel Syndrome often experience problems with gripping and might notice the signs of muscle atrophy.

The best way to try and prevent the muscles from continuing to weaken is to use some form of grip strengthener. It is a good idea to buy a couple of different strengtheners as they often work in different ways and will offer different methods of challenging the muscles, which will help to avoid overusing the same muscles.

Exercise balls are suitable for most people and are comfortable to use. These could be used in conjunction with a piece of equipment to strengthen the hands and fingers.

To get the most from the strengthening exercises, try a protein powder to help build and feed the muscles

When exercising, remember to gently warm the muscles first and stretch them out afterwards.

Sufferer's story: *"I've ...spent money on prescriptions, osteos, ice/ heat packs, massagers, VR software, microphones, acupuncture, Alexander technique lessons etc so we must be talking £3000 plus. I had to work part time for a few months in 2001 because I was ill so I lost around £2,400 in income that year. I've just spent extra money on an automatic car so it's less pressure on my hands so that's another extra cost. I've been lucky though and kept working so I've been able to afford these things. I can't see that someone on sick/ disability pay could."* Source: Watson, M. 2009. Investigating the experiences of people with RSI. http://etheses.qmu.ac.uk/133/
Care Grants, and others.

5) Splinting and Taping

Splinting or taping the affected wrist will give the area some support and reduce the strain on other areas of the body such as the shoulders, that often end up being overused when there is a weakness lower down in the arm.

A GP or consultant can refer a patient to a physio, and they will decide if they feel splints would be suitable.

While it is not advisable, if you do decide to buy your own splints, don't buy ones that are too rigid as they can often hold the hands too tense and cause pain in the shoulders.

If it is suggested that you wear splints for actions such as typing or using a till, be sure to take the splints off regularly and stretch your hands and fingers out or they tend to end up feeling cramped and tight.

Sports tape is a good idea for people that just want some light support. Remember to leave a gap on the palm side when applying the tape and stretch the wrist out regularly throughout the day so the muscles don't tighten up.

6) Occupational Therapists and Workplace Ergonomics

This book explains the role of occupational therapists and how they can help patients with Carpal Tunnel Syndrome manage their symptoms. Occupational therapists can offer help and advice for finding a better work position to help lessen the impact on the hands and wrists.

An occupational therapist can also suggest useful gadgets that can be used around the home to make everyday tasks easier.

7) Ergonomic work equipment

Ergonomic work equipment is readily available now and tools can be obtained for almost any occupation or hobby to reduce the strain on the wrists.

8) Leisure Time and Sleep

It is not unusual for people to have an occupation that requires a lot of repetitive work, and then to go home and either continue their work into the evening or indulge in hobbies such as game playing.

In addition, many people have a poor sleeping posture, and all of this combined can lead to an almost constant strain on the wrists.

Look at your schedule and see how you can do things differently and if you wake up in the morning with a lot of pain, you need to make some alterations to your sleeping posture, such as propping yourself up on a cushion so that you don't roll over and sleep on your affected wrist or use memory foam products for better support when you rest.

Sufferer's story: *"I was 22 and working as a legal secretary when I first felt pain in my arms. I ignored it, thinking or hoping it would go away, and continued to work at my normal pace. I had recently changed jobs and didn't want to cause any problems. However, typing for six or seven hours a day I soon realised the pain was getting worse. I continued working for about six months then my employer put me off work. It got to the stage that I couldn't type more than a few minutes at a time and couldn't keep up with the workload. They didn't have any light duties for me nor did they want to re-instate me unless I could type as much as I had previously. In the end, they legally terminated my employment after I had been off work for six months." Source: RSI and Overuse Injury Association of the ACT*

9) Paying Attention to Emotions

For most people, CTS brings up a torrent of emotions. People fear losing their livelihoods, relationships and enjoyment of life. They may see their independence, financial security, and ability to deal with daily life slipping away. It's understandable that they would be upset, angry, depressed, or afraid.

Depression has many faces. You may feel sad, cry easily, and feel helpless. You may have difficulty sleeping, or sleep too much. You may feel guilty, ashamed, or bad about yourself. You may eat more or less, gain weight or lose it. You may become irritable, impatient, or unreasonable without knowing it. Impotence or lack of interest in sex may accompany depression. Friendships may slip away as you isolate yourself. You may use drugs or alcohol to try to relieve the depression—but they only make things worse.

Accepting your injury and the limitations it poses is an important step toward recovery. Acceptance gives your permission to ask for and receive help, starting the process of recovery. The Persian poet Rumi wrote: "If you desire healing, let yourself fall ill."

Feelings can be uncomfortable, especially if you are not used to paying attention to them. You may think having feelings is a sign of weakness, but the truth is that dealing with your emotions is essential to healing. Our emotions are a big part of who we are; we can try to ignore them, or we can learn more about them and use them to support our recovery.

Taking care of your emotions means finding someone you can talk to openly without worrying about judgment or repercussions. That could be a trusted friend, a spiritual counsellor, a support group, or a professional psychotherapist. A medical professional, like a psychiatrist, psychotherapist, or general practitioner, can help you develop a treatment plan for the depression. You may decide to take medication as part of your treatment plan. The plan may include taking depression medications as well as making changes in your outlook and lifestyle.

A positive attitude, hard as that may seem, aids recovery from depression. Treat yourself kindly, with compassion--as you would a friend who is in pain. Focus on your progress, on small improvements in functioning and pain relief. Stay active, finding hobbies or volunteer work that you enjoy. A repetitive strain injury may limit your activities, but it doesn't eliminate all activities.

10) Asking for Help

Many people find that they need more help with daily activities than they did before. It seems that the more we need help, the harder it is to ask for it. While we may not hesitate to help a friend, we may feel uncomfortable asking that same friend for help.

Here are some ideas to make asking easier:

- Take advantage of help that you may not have accepted in the past. For example, say yes when the grocery bagger offers to carry your sacks to your car, or pull up to a petrol station that has attendants to pump for you.

- If you are able to pay for services that will make life easier for you. Send out the ironing and pay a cleaning service to change the bedding and hoover, it will be easier to tend to tasks only you can do, like taking care of your children or performing well on your job or playing a round of golf with a friend.

- Barter for help. Maybe a teenager in the neighbourhood will mow your lawn in exchange for help with schoolwork. Or you could babysit a friend's child whilst the friend does the marketing for both of you.

Ask for what you need on the job. If you need more breaks or a different chair, work with your boss to arrange it. It's difficult to ask at work but if you don't you may not be able to work at all. Remember, it's to your employer's benefit to keep you safe on the job. A good employer will want to know what you need and how to accommodate it.

Conclusion

You've read it all, you've read the sufferer's stories. Surely you do NOT want to be one of these sufferers. You don't need to be.

Therefore you MUST pay attention to your own health. Your office environment, your mobile phone, your game console, your laptop are NOT safe for your health unless YOU make them safe by taking breaks and doing regular exercises.

In my opinion, all electronic devices from this modern society should have pop-up software on that throws messages at the user like "get off this computer" or "stop texting" or "time for exercises".

I have break-software on my computer and I urge everybody to do the same. The software I use is: www.breakremindersoftware.com **(only available for PC, not for Mac)** and in my opinion this should be installed on each computer that is sold anywhere in the world. The software monitors the time you work on the computer and it alerts you when you need to take a break. You can set it to block your keyboard during breaks so you cannot work. You can choose to override your settings should you wish to do so but I suggest you set them as "Whatever I do, give me a break". My settings are as follows:

- I have a break for 20 seconds every 10 minutes and I've set the software so that my keyboard is blocked. Therefore every 10 minutes I do some gentle neck and arm exercises.

- I have a 10-minute break every hour and my software is set so my keyboard is blocked, which forces me to get up and do something else for 10 minutes.

If you can afford it, invest in www.breakremindersoftware.com. It is the best piece of software available for an office environment.

You have been warned: install it as a matter of urgency if you can afford it.

If you cannot afford it: force yourself to take regular breaks.

I do realise that some of the ergonomic furniture and aids pictured or talked about in this book are expensive but if you can, drink a few cups of coffee less per month or reduce your alcohol consumption and buy some of the aids to prevent RSI in your life.

I end this book with the message I've put at the beginning:

It is no joke, really, please take this seriously and look after your future health.

Don't ignore your symptoms as it really comes down to this one simple message:

ACT NOW

OR

SUFFER FOREVER!

Vendors of Equipment and Software for Prevention

A growing number of manufacturers produce ergonomically designed equipment. The following list of vendors represent only a small percentage of those that sell software and equipment that can help prevent RSIs and improve conditions for those recovering from repetitive strain injuries.

Inclusion in this list or in the text of this book does not indicate endorsement of products or vendors, nor does absence from the list indicate lack of approval. Many products billed as ergonomically designed are not effective in preventing RSIs; buyers need to study the products carefully to see if they meet their needs.

Software

Break Reminder Software

www.breakremindersoftware.com

www.workpace.com

www.rsiprevention.com

www.rsiguard.com

Computer User Exercise Software

AtTheDeskSoftware www.atthedesksoftware.com

Voice Recognition Software

Dragon Naturally Speaking www.dragonvoicerecognition.com

TalkingDesktop www.talkingdesktop.com

Equipment

Alternative Workstations

Anthro (www.Anthro.com)

Ergo Desk (www.ErgoDesk.com)

Ergolcd.com (http://www.ergolcd.com/)

Ergotron (www.ergotron.com)

GeekDesk (www.geekdesk.com/)

Nielsen http://www.nielsen-associates.co.uk/sit-stand

Steelcase (http://www.steelcase.com)

Treadmill Desk (www.treadmill-desk.com/)

Chairs

Herman Miller
(http://www.hermanmiller.com/products/seating.html)

Sit4Less (www.sit4less.com/)

Alternative Keyboards

ErgonomicKeyboards www.ergonomickeyboards.org

FrogPad www.frogpad.com

Keytools www.keytools.co.uk/keyboards

Source 1 Ergonomics. www.source1ergonomics.com

Alternative Mice and Other Pointing Devices

Amazon.com www.amazon.co.uk/Foot-Mouse-Slipper-Programmable-Pedal/dp/B0061DVAOK

FrogPad (www.frogpad.com)

Gizmag www.gizmag.com

Keytools www.keytools.com/mice

Liberator www.liberator.co.uk/headmouse-extreme.html

Price Selector (http://uk.price-selector.net/search/foot%20pedal%20mouse?campid=5336926831)

Source 1 Ergonomics http://www.source1ergonomics.com

Techcess http://www.techcess.co.uk/5_1_headmouse.php

The Human Solution www.thehumansolution.com/mice.html

Laptop Carrying Cases

BBP Bags http://www.bbpbags.com

Bizrate http://www.bizrate.co.uk

Mobile Phones for Children

Fireflyhttp://www.fireflymobile.com

Teddyfone www.kiddyfone.com

Workstation Equipment for Children

Ask Ergo Works, Inc.http://www.askergoworks.com

Chester Creek Technologies http://www.chestercreektech.com

Tiny Einsteins Computer Products http://www.tinyeinsteins.com

QWERTY Keyboard, Computer Keyboards for Children
www.qwertykeyboard.org

Aids for Daily Living

Assistive Devices Key
(http://www.assistivedeviceskey.com/category/891098)

Great Grips (http://www.greatgrips.com)

Oxo Good Grips. (www.oxo.com)

Life with Ease (http://www.lifewithease.com/

Websites for More Information

Claims Management Company. www.antriumlegal.com

American Horticultural Therapy Association. www.ahta.org

British Chiropractic Association. http://www.chiropractic-uk.co.uk/

Canadian Centre for Occupational Health and Safety. http://www.ccohs.ca/oshanswers/ergonomics/office/stretching.html

Canadian Horticultural Therapy Association. www.chta.ca

Chartered Institute of Personnel and Development (CIPD). http://www.cipd.co.uk/hr-resources/practical-tools/absence-management.aspx

CTD News. www.ctdnew.com

Department for Work and Pensions. http://www.dwp.gov.uk/fitnote/

Ergomatters. www.ergomatters.co.uk.

Ergonomics-Info.com. http://www.ergonomics-info.com/index.html

European Agency for Workplace Safety and Health. http://osha.europa.eu/en/campaigns/ew2007/

Health and Safety Executive. http://www.hse.gov.uk/msd/index.htm

International Ergonomics Association. http://www.iea.cc/ECEE/guidelines.html

Kids Health.
http://kidshealth.org/parent/firstaid_safe/home/ergonomics.html

Mayo Clinic. www.mayoclinic.com

Forum where pain sufferers can get help from fellow sufferers.
There are people on this forum who have cured RSI using mind
body techniques www.tmshelp.com.

National Health Service (NHS).
www.nhs.uk/conditions/repetitive-strain-injury/

National Institute for Occupational Safety and Health (NIOSH).
http://www.cdc.gov/niosh

Public and Commercial Services Union.
http://www.pcs.org.uk/en/resources/health_and_safety/guide_to_r
epetitive_strain_injury.cfm

RSI Action: The National Repetitive Strain Injury Charity.
http://www.rsiaction.org.uk/

RSI and Overuse Injury Association of the ACT.
http://www.rsi.org.au/index.html

RSI Help. http://www.rsihelp.com/

RSI Treatment Blog. http://rsitreatmentblog.com/cgi-
sys/suspendedpage.cgi.

RSI-UK. www.rsi-uk.org.uk

Trellis: Supporting Health through Horticulture.
http://www.trellisscotland.org.uk/

Typing Injury FAQ. http://www.tifaq.org

United States Department of Labor/Occupational Safety & Health Administration (OSHA). http://www.osha.gov/SLTC/etools/computerworkstations/

Working-Well. http://www.working-well.org/

Finding Suppliers

All of the products detailed in this book are available online.

Ergonomic products such as a mouse for carpal tunnel syndrome can be purchased from specialist stores. If you cannot find a specialist store that delivers to your area, then all of the products detailed in chapter five can be brought from Amazon.

Carpal Tunnel gloves that provide light compression to the area are readily available and specialist sport stores all stock a variety of carpal tunnel wrist supports or wrist splints for the carpal tunnel area.

The vitamins and supplements listed in this book can all be purchased from health shops either online or offline. If there are problems finding any of the items, then they are readily available via Amazon and eBay.

Carpal Tunnel Supports and Carpal Tunnel braces are available from specialist sports stores. If there is difficulty obtaining them in your local area, then online stores such as Amazon and eBay have a large range of these products available for delivery.

Support Groups

It is always good to share experiences and tips with others that suffer from Carpal Tunnel Syndrome. Sometimes all people need is somebody that understands what they are feeling and how their condition is affecting them.

In support groups, people talk about their own experiences as well as sharing hints and advice. Visitors to the support groups can also read about other people's experiences of surgery and get recommendations for the best Carpal Tunnel splints and braces, find different ways of managing pain, or just find someone to talk to.

People are only too keen to share their tips on how to relieve their symptoms of Carpal Tunnel Syndrome and how they alleviate their symptoms or natural remedies for Carpal Tunnel Syndrome.

Forums can be very encouraging as people often share their experiences of their carpal tunnel recovery and share ideas for carpal tunnel exercises to help reduce symptoms.

Listed in this section are some support groups that are available online:

Daily Strength Carpal Tunnel Syndrome Support Group

This forum is updated regularly and there are always plenty of discussions underway. Anyone can sign up and participate or just read the posts and gain knowledge from other users of the group.

There are all sorts of useful discussions such as finding the right wrist brace for Carpal Tunnel Syndrome or the correct wrist support brace. Patients also discuss how carpal tunnel decompression surgery has worked for them and effective ways that they have found of treating carpal tunnel problems.

http://www.dailystrength.org/c/Carpal-Tunnel-Syndrome/support-group

MDJunction

The MDJunction website has a forum dedicated to Carpal Tunnel Syndrome sufferers. The forum is usually very active and as well as learning about other people's experiences of Carpal Tunnel Syndrome, there are also discussions about Cubital Tunnel Syndrome.

There are plenty of posts about finding effective Carpal Tunnel wrist splints or Carpal Tunnel braces and people also discus Carpal Tunnel surgery and Carpal Tunnel remedies.

http://www.mdjunction.com/carpal-tunnel-syndrome

Carpal Tunnel Syndrome Support Group

Members can get advice on finding the right kind of carpal tunnel syndrome braces, read about people's experiences with surgery and find out how other people cope with the different symptoms of Carpal Tunnel Syndrome.

The forum can be found at: http://carpal-tunnel-syndrome.supportgroups.com/

eHealth Forum

The eHealth Forum is another good community that is full of useful advice for patients with Carpal Tunnel Syndrome. There are plenty of discussions such as the various types of Carpal Tunnel Syndrome surgery, after effects of the surgery, carpal tunnel pain relief, dealing with pain, finding wrist splints for Carpal Tunnel Syndrome, and managing the symptoms.

http://ehealthforum.com/health/carpal_tunnel_syndrome.html

Inspire.com

Inspire.com has forums for many different health conditions, including Carpal Tunnel Syndrome. Visitors have to sign up to the forum before they can view any of the discussions on the site or contribute to any of the discussions.

https://www.inspire.com/conditions/carpal-tunnel-syndrome/

Health Tap

Health Tap is a forum with a difference. People can post a question on the forum and get free advice from a US-based doctor. Many of the doctors contributing to this site specialise in hand surgery so if a patient has some questions about their surgery and they haven't thought to ask their own doctors, then this site is a valuable resource.

The site can be found by going to:
https://www.healthtap.com/topics/carpal-tunnel-syndrome-support-groups

National Association of Injured and Disabled Workers

The association is based in the United States, but the site can be accessed by anyone no matter what their location. They have forums for a range of medical conditions that affect US workers, and they also have a board that is dedicated to Carpal Tunnel Syndrome.

Users are invited to contribute to the site and share their experiences. The forum can be found by going to:
https://www.naidw.org/forum/131-carpal-tunnel-syndrome/261-carpal-tunnel-syndrome-support-group

Resources

Access to work grants are available for residents in the UK if they are trying to get back to work, need assistance to stay in work, or if they are self-employed.

These grants do not have to be paid back and the amount that a person is entitled to will vary according to their needs. Access to work funding can be used to help pay for the equipment needed in order to stay in work. For instance, it can cover the cost of workplace adaptations and for the cost of specialist equipment.

To qualify for the grant, applicants must be aged over 16 and live in England or Wales, be in work, or about the start work, and their disability or illness must affect their ability to do their job.

These grants can also be given to employers to cover the cost of any workplace adaptations that need to be made. For instance, if you need to use voice activated software, need to use an ergonomic chair, or need to change your work station so it is ergonomically sound.

Details of these grants can be found by going to:

https://www.gov.uk/access-to-work/how-to-claim

Carpal Tunnel Syndrome Exercises

Video tuitions featuring exercises for Carpal Tunnel Syndrome are available online:

Demonstrations of Carpal Tunnel Syndrome treatment exercises are available at the following links:

http://www.youtube.com/watch?v=I5RHbdRcmvA

http://www.youtube.com/watch?v=MwGPgXL5QLU

Massage techniques to help reduce the symptoms of Carpal Tunnel Syndrome:

http://www.youtube.com/watch?v=9PMb2fnJ1Zg

Carpal Tunnel Syndrome and Pregnancy video:

http://www.nhs.uk/Video/Pages/carpal-tunnel-syndrome-animation.asp

Glossary

Carpal Tunnel

A narrow tunnel inside the wrist

Carpal Tunnel Syndrome:

 An entrapment of the median nerve

Cubital Tunnel Syndrome

A compression of the ulna nerve

Endoscopic surgery

During endoscopic surgery, small cuts will be made into the body and an endoscope used to examine the cause of a patient's symptoms.

EMG

An electromyogram will help diagnose nerve problems such as tarsal and carpal tunnel syndrome

Epicondylitis

When the tendons that cover the epicondyle in the elbow area become inflamed, this is known as Epicondylitis or tennis elbow.

Glenohumeral joint

The shoulder joint

Golfer's Elbow

See Epicondylitis

Humerus

A bone in the upper arm

Hypothyroid

A person with low levels of thyroid will be described as having hypothyroidism

Motor

The motor nerves carry impulses from the spinal cord or brain.

Nerve conduction studies

Nerve conduction studies examine how well the nerves are firing and how fast.

Neuropathy

A disease affecting the nerves

Osteopathy

Gentle, hands on technique to help mobilise the body and heal aches and pains.

Sensory

Sensory nerves carry impulses from the peripheral (hands and Feet) to the nervous system

Tinel's test

The Tinel's Test is used to confirm the diagnosis of Carpal Tunnel Syndrome. The physician will tap the median nerve and if it causes symptoms such as tingling or pain in the fingers then it will be considered a positive sign that a patient has CTS

Trigger point massage

When touched, trigger points will cause pain in the body. Using trigger point massage can help to relieve this discomfort

Further Reading

Conquering Carpal Tunnel Syndrome and Other Repetitive Strain Injuries Butler, Sharon J.

The Carpal Tunnel Helpbook, Fried, Scott

The Natural Treatment of Carpal Tunnel Syndrome, Wunderlich Jr Ray C.

Carpal Tunnel Syndrome Solution, McCloud, Ace

Fixing You: Shoulder and Elbow Pain, Oldrman, Rick

RSI and how to avoid it, Cope Bowley, Tonia

Trigger Point Therapy for Repetitive Strain Injury: Your Self-Treatment Workbook for Elbow, Lower Arm, Wrist, & Hand Pain, DeLaune, Valerie

The Posture Workbook: Free Yourself from Back, Neck and Shoulder Pain with the Alexander Technique, Nicholls, Carolyn

DVDs

Say goodbye to wrist pain: Wrist pain Therapy

The Natural Way Pain Free Shoulder, Elbow and Wrist pain – Andrea Metcalf

Stretch Away Wrist Pain

Stretch away muscle pain at your desk

Clinical Trigger Point Therapy Protocol for Hand and Wrist Pain

Healthy Hands, Wrists and Forearms

Acknowledgements

Special thanks to Nathan Wei, M.D. from the
www.arthritistreatmentcenter.com

And Debbie Amini, occupational therapist.

Thanks to my family for supporting me in whatever I do.

Sources

Acupuncture in patients with carpal tunnel syndrome: A randomized controlled trial.

Yang CP, Hsieh CL, Wang NH, Li TC, Hwang KL, Yu SC, Chang MH.

Yoga-based Intervention for Carpal Tunnel Syndrome

Marian S. Garfinkel, EdD; Atul Singhal, MD; Warren A. Katz, MD; David A. Allan, MD, PhD; Rosemary Reshetar, EdD; H. Ralph Schumacher, Jr, MD

The carpal tunnel syndrome is a bilateral disorder

A. E. Bagatur, G. Zorer

From SSK Istanbul Training Hospital, Turkey

Omega-3 fatty acids for neuropathic pain: case series

Ko GD, Nowacki NB, Arseneau L, Eitel M, Hum A.

Carpal tunnel syndrome and vitamin B6.

Ryan-Harshman M, Aldoori W.

Amelioration by mecobalamin of subclinical carpal tunnel syndrome involving unaffected limbs in stroke patients.

Sato Y, Honda Y, Iwamoto J, Kanoko T, Satoh K.

Vitamin B6, vitamin C, and carpal tunnel syndrome. A cross-sectional study of 441 adults

Keniston RC, Nathan PA, Leklem JE, Lockwood RS

Treatment of carpal tunnel syndrome with alpha-lipoic acid

Sources

Di Geronimo G, Caccese AF, Caruso L, Soldati A, Passaretti U.

Use of Arnica to relieve pain after carpal-tunnel release surgery.

Jeffrey SL, Belcher HJ.

EMLA cream for carpal tunnel syndrome: how it compares with steroid injection.

Moghtaderi AR, Jazayeri SM, Azizi S.

Ultrasound-Guided Percutaneous Injection, Hydrodissection and Fenestration for Carpal Tunnel Syndrome: Description of a new technique

Daniel G, Malone, M.D., Thomas B. Clark, DC, RVT

Nathan Wei, MD

Published by IMB Publishing 2014

Copyright and Trademarks. This publication is Copyright 2014 by IMB Publishing. All products, publications, software and services mentioned and recommended in this publication are protected by trademarks. In such instance, all trademarks & copyright belong to the respective owners. All rights reserved. No part of this book may be reproduced or transferred in any form or by any means, graphic, electronic, or mechanical, including photocopying, recording, taping, or by any information storage retrieval system, without the written permission of the author. Pictures used in this book are either royalty free pictures bought from stock-photo websites or have the source mentioned underneath the picture. Disclaimer and Legal Notice. This product is not legal or medical advice and should not be interpreted in that manner. You need to do your own due-diligence to determine if the content of this product is right for you. The author and the affiliates of this product are not liable for any damages or losses associated with the content in this product. While every attempt has been made to verify the information shared in this publication, neither the author nor the affiliates assume any responsibility for errors, omissions or contrary interpretation of the subject matter herein. Any perceived slights to any specific person(s) or organization(s) are purely unintentional. We have no control over the nature, content and availability of the web sites listed in this book. The inclusion of any web site links does not necessarily imply a recommendation or endorse the views expressed within them. IMB Publishing takes no responsibility for, and will not be liable for, the websites being temporarily unavailable or being removed from the internet. The accuracy and completeness of information provided herein and opinions stated herein are not guaranteed or warranted to produce any particular results, and the advice and strategies, contained herein may not be suitable for every individual. The author shall not be liable for any loss incurred as a consequence of the use and application, directly or indirectly, of any information presented in this work. This publication is designed to provide information in regards to the subject matter covered. The information included in this book has been compiled to give an overview of carpal tunnel syndrome and detail some of the symptoms, treatments etc. that are available to people with this condition. It is not intended to give medical advice. For a firm diagnosis of your condition, and for a treatment plan suitable for you, you should consult your doctor or consultant. The writer of this book and the publisher are not responsible for any damages or negative consequences following any of the treatments or methods highlighted in this book. Website links are for informational purposes and should not be seen as a personal endorsement; the same applies to the products detailed in this book.

www.ingramcontent.com/pod-product-compliance
Lightning Source LLC
Chambersburg PA
CBHW060548200326
41521CB00007B/529